Surviving
Prostate
Cancer

Surviving Prostate Cancer

What You Need to Know
to Make Informed Decisions

E. FULLER TORREY, M.D.

Illustrations by Carlton Stoiber

YALE UNIVERSITY PRESS / NEW HAVEN & LONDON

The information and suggestions contained in this book are not intended to replace the services of your physician or caregiver. Because each person and each medical situation is unique, you should consult your own physician to get answers to your personal questions, to evaluate any symptoms you may have, or to receive suggestions on appropriate medications.

The author has attempted to make this book as accurate and up-to-date as possible, but it may nevertheless contain errors, omissions, or material that is out-of-date at the time you read it. Neither the author nor the publisher has any legal responsibility or liability for errors, omissions, out-of-date material, or the reader's application of the medical information or advice contained in this book.

Quotations of Anatole Broyard are from *Intoxicated by My Illness,* copyright © 1992 by the Estate of Anatole Broyard. Used by permission of Clarkson Potter/Publishers, a division of Random House, Inc.

Designed by Mary Valencia.
Set in Stone type by Keystone Typesetting, Inc.
Printed in the United States of America.

The Library of Congress has cataloged the hardcover edition as follows:
Torrey, E. Fuller (Edwin Fuller), 1937–
Surviving prostate cancer: what you need to know to make informed
decisions / E. Fuller Torrey.
p. cm. — (Yale University Press health & wellness)
Includes bibliographical references (p.).
ISBN-13: 978-0-300-11640-3 (alk. paper)
ISBN-10: 0-300-11640-3 (alk. paper)
1. Prostate—Cancer—Treatment—Popular works. 2. Prostate—Cancer—Popular works. I. Title. II. Series.
RC280.P7T67 2006
616.99'463—dc22   2006044726

ISBN 978-0-300-12607-5 (pbk. : alk. paper)

A catalogue record for this book is available from the British Library.

The paper in this book meets the guidelines for permanence and durability of the Committee on Production Guidelines for Book Longevity of the Council on Library Resources.

10 9 8 7 6 5 4 3 2 1

For Barbara, my partner for four decades,
who has been exceptional in good times
and extraordinary in bad times

C O N T E N T S

ACKNOWLEDGMENTS

I am deeply indebted to Dr. Michael Newman, my internist and friend, and to Dr. Nicholas Constantinople, my urologist. Dr. Newman detected my cancer while my PSA (prostate specific antigen) was within normal limits and, with luck, still curable. Dr. Constantinople's kindness is exceeded only by his surgical skills. I would not wish prostate cancer on any man, but I would hope that anyone who is affected could have access to two such fine physicians.

Dr. Constantinople also provided useful comments on the manuscript, as did Halsey Beemer, Lew Bigelow, Stephen Hersh, Bob McGee, Brad Northrup, David Robinson, Michael Viola, and Isaiah Zimmerman. The book was much improved by their many suggestions.

I am grateful to Carlton Stoiber for contributing the excellent drawings and cartoons, thereby raising the book to a significantly higher level.

Several people responded readily to my queries, including Christina Duenas, David Miller, Alan Partin, and Thomas Stamey. Richard Atkins and Monica Alexander at the National Prostate Cancer Coalition and David McLeod and Jane Hudak at the Center for Prostate Disease Research were generous with their time and knowledge. In addition, I gratefully acknowledge the following:

Gordon Sheppard, for permission to quote from "The Wondrous World of Prostate Cancer," an unpublished essay;

Geoff Barnard, for permission to quote from a private letter;

Mark Litwin, for permission to reprint the UCLA Prostate Cancer Index for Urinary Function;

Michael Dorso, for permission to quote from his *Seeds of Hope;*

Patricia Zline and Madison Books, for permission to quote from *Adam's Burden,* by Charles Neider;

The Estate of Anatole Broyard and Random House, Inc., for permission to quote from Broyard's *Intoxicated by My Illness*.

I am especially indebted to Jean Black, Senior Editor at Yale University Press, for believing in the book despite a plethora of other prostate books on the market. It has been a pleasure to work with her, as well as with Laura Davulis, Jessie Hunnicutt, and Margaret Otzel. The book was also much improved by the careful editing of Vivian Wheeler.

Judy Miller was once again a superb research assistant, fact checker, typist, and kind enforcer of correct grammar; the book is much better because of her help.

Most important, I am indebted to Halsey Beemer, Stephen Hersh, Robert Taylor, Sidney Wolfe, Bob Yolken, and other friends for their encouragement, and especially to Barbara Torrey for all of the above and more, much more. Being diagnosed with cancer is a defining experience, especially defining of one's supporters.

ABBREVIATIONS

BMI   body mass index

BPH   benign prostatic hypertrophy

CT   computerized tomography

DES   diethylstilbestrol

DHT   dihydrotestosterone

DRE   digital rectal exam

EBRT   external beam radiation therapy

EORTC   European Organization for Research and Treatment of Cancer

HDR   high dose rate brachytherapy

HIFU   high-intensity focused ultrasound

HMO   Health Maintenance Organization

HPV   human papillomavirus

IMRT   intensity-modulated radiotherapy

LH   luteinizing hormone

LHRH   luteinizing hormone-release hormone

LSN   lymphotrophic superparamagnetic nanoparticles

MRI   magnetic resonance imaging

NCI   National Cancer Institute

PC   prostate cancer

PCF   Prostate Cancer Foundation

PIN   prostatic intraepithelial neoplasia

PIVOT   Prostate Cancer Intervention Versus Observation Trial

PLCO   Prostate, Lung, Colorectal and Ovarian Cancer Screening Trial

PSA   prostate specific antigen

RTOG   Radiation Therapy Group

SELECT   Selenium and Vitamin E Cancer Prevention Trial

STD   sexually transmitted disease

3DCRT   three-dimensional conformal radiation therapy

TNM   tumor, node, metastasis staging system to describe whether the cancer has spread

Surviving
Prostate
Cancer

1

On Being Diagnosed

I n the timeline of our memories, major tragedies stand out as spikes. Most people remember clearly what they were doing when they learned that hijacked airliners had crashed into the World Trade Center. Those of us who are old enough can pinpoint precisely where we were when we heard that President Kennedy had been shot. Being diagnosed with prostate cancer is comparable.

I was sitting at my desk at the Stanley Medical Research Institute at 10 A.M. on May 4, 2004. The immediate problem was how to persuade research staff members who do not like one another to work together. I was not expecting the call, because my urologist had said the pathology report after my biopsy would take seven to ten days to compile, and this was only day six.

The arrival of the call did not unduly alarm me—at first—because I was reasonably certain that the lump in my prostate was benign and the biopsy would be negative. My prostate specific antigen (PSA) was only 3.3, well within the normal range, and the urologist had not seen any suspicious-looking areas on ultrasound at the time of the biopsy. Besides, I was a healthy 66 years old and planning to live at least twenty more years. I had only recently acquired a few harbingers of old age: forgetting names, a diminished urinary stream, and plaques on the skin. And I hadn't yet passed the definitive landmark

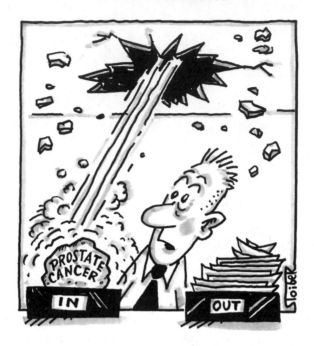

of the aged: sending obituaries of old friends to other old friends. Cancer was not something I was supposed to get; cancer was for other people. As one man put it: "Prostate cancer was as remote from the possibilities I imagined for myself as a voyage to the moon."[1]

The urologist did not preface it as "bad news," but announced in a straightforward way that the biopsy had been positive, that I had cancer in three of the nine cores (samples) taken during the biopsy, and that the Gleason score was 7. In an effort to wrap my mind around this meteor that had just broken through the roof and landed on my desk, I asked what the Gleason score meant. The only Gleason I knew was old-time comedian Jackie Gleason, but I doubted he had anything to do with prostate cancer. I also wondered to myself why I had not done any reading on prostate cancer, so that I could interpret Gleason scores and numbers of positive cores, but then remembered that I had been virtually certain I didn't have it, so why waste my time?

A Gleason 7, he said, was an "intermediate" stage of cancer. It meant that the cells were not as benign as a Gleason 4, 5, or 6 but not as malignant as an 8, 9, or 10. I did not like the sound of

An Unwelcome Surprise

When my doctor said, "General, you have prostate cancer," I was thrust into an immediate and fearful state of confusion. I can still recall my inability to move a muscle for what seemed like an eternity after hearing my diagnosis.

—Gen. H. Norman Schwarzkopf
U.S. Army, retired

"I have cancer?"

"Yes. In the left lobe."

"So now, at last, I *know*," I thought, and my ground-floor study, surrounded on three sides by a yard and trees, in which I had taken his call, seemed to darken. "Everything has changed. From now on cancer isn't *out there*. It's the enemy *inside me*, eating away at something vital." I experienced the cliché sinking feeling, as if something had suddenly happened to my blood pressure.

—Charles Neider, *Adam's Burden*

"intermediate"; it reminded me of the *C* I had gotten in intermediate algebra. I also remembered all too clearly from my histology course in medical school what "intermediate" cancer cells looked like under a microscope. They were ugly and misshapen, not as bad as the grossly deformed cells that would qualify as Gleason 9 or 10, but certainly not to be confused with normal, orderly-looking cells. And the urologist was telling me that the ugly cells were inside *me*, now, as I sat at my desk. Unbelievable. I was deeply resentful and felt that I had been surreptitiously violated.

The remainder of the workday had an illusory quality. I called my wife, but said nothing to anyone else. I needed first to understand the news myself. My strongest memories of the day are of listening to other people complain about things and being sorely tempted to cut them off, saying, "Why are *you* complaining, *I've* got cancer!" In the late afternoon, I listened as a research colleague wallowed in his personal and professional woes for almost an hour. I wondered briefly whether, if I strangled him, a jury would find me not guilty because of mitigating circumstances. Then, driving home, I got caught in the worst traffic jam I had encountered in months. Sitting there, I thought of Job. "Man is born to trouble, as the sparks fly upward," it was written. This had to be the archetypal bad day.

My immediate task was to learn as much as I could about prostate cancer and my options for treatment. I realized that I, a trained physician, knew almost nothing about the prostate. It appeared to be, in fact, the most obscure and least interesting organ in the body. In anatomy class, my group of four students had had a female cadaver to dissect, while the group at the next table had had a male. Our instructor had told us to change tables periodically so that we would understand the anatomy of both sexes. It hadn't happened. Our almost all-male class had a personal as well as a professional interest in female anatomy and, more often than not, eight of us were working at our table. I'm not sure I even saw a prostate.

How long did I have to make a decision? One book on prostate cancer advised you to "commit to a therapeutic strategy within about three to six months after you're diagnosed," but sooner if your cancer is "large and high grade." One study reported that delays in treatment of more than three months increased chances of recurrence ten years later. Another study found that prostate cancers for which treatment was begun an average of two months after diagnosis did not have an increase in recurrence three years later. A large 2005 study was the most reassuring, finding that surgical delays of up to a year after biopsy did not increase chances of recurrence five years later; therefore, "men who wait several months after biopsy before undergoing RP [surgery] are not jeopardizing their probability of cure."[2] This lack of professional consensus on important prostate cancer issues would, I would soon discover, turn out to be common.

In general, I am neither laid back nor indecisive, and I found that with cancer growing inside of me, all sense of leisure disappeared. Despite reported assurances that prostate cancer is slow growing, I heard only the word *growing*, not the word *slow*. Each day that passed meant that my cancer had grown, and perhaps spread. One day it

---

A New Land

I sensed that I had crossed some invisible line into a new phase of my life, the way a traveler might feel when crossing a frontier and entering a different country, with a strange language, new customs, different rules, signs that made no sense, policemen with unfamiliar uniforms pacing in pairs up and down the railway platforms.

Michael Korda, *Man to Man*

---

would be contained within the prostate gland and perhaps curable, but there would come a day when it would not be. Which day would that be?

It seemed obvious that the thing I needed most was accurate information. I found myself identifying with retired general Norman Schwarzkopf, who, on being diagnosed with prostate cancer, said: "For me it was like war. First thing you do is learn about the enemy."[3] As a researcher, I had dozens of questions I wanted answered, taking into consideration all available studies. As a person with cancer, I wanted them all answered yesterday.

My search of books and professional papers told me that, according to the American Cancer Society, I was one of 230,110 men in 2004 who were being diagnosed with prostate cancer. Discouragingly, that number had not changed much in recent years. It meant that 630 men were being diagnosed every day, 26 every hour, 1 every 2.3 minutes, Sundays and holidays included. Two hundred thirty thousand, one hundred ten men is equivalent to the entire male and female population of Danbury, Connecticut, or Olympia, Washington. I had been in Danbury and Olympia, and that seemed like a lot of people. I also learned that 1.6 million American men currently have, or have had, prostate cancer—which is more than the metropolitan population of Columbus, Memphis, Milwaukee, Sacramento, or San Antonio. Misery loves company, but having all that company didn't make me feel any better.

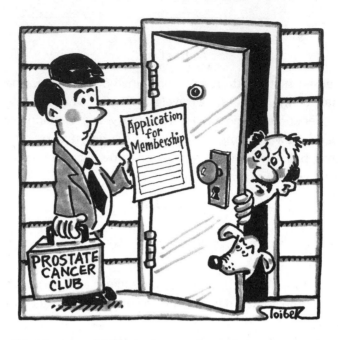

"No, the man of the house is *not* at home."

My reading also informed me that I had joined the ranks of some notable men who have had prostate cancer, including athletes such as Stan Musial, Arnold Palmer, and Len Dawson, and political leaders such as Bob Dole and Rudy Giuliani. Even Andrew von Eschenbach, director of the National Cancer Institute from 2002 to 2005, has had prostate cancer, and that didn't seem promising. All these men were members of the Prostate Cancer Club. Joining such a club provided little consolation—good grief, I had not even applied for membership. I was even more discouraged by the list of former club members, now deceased. It included educated, important, and wealthy men with access to the best available medical resources. The most disheartening name on the list was that of Willet Whitmore, who had been chief of urology at Memorial Sloan-Kettering Cancer Center and regarded as one of the nation's experts on prostate cancer.

Ultimately, my search for information about prostate cancer was disappointing on three counts. First, I was appalled to learn how little was known with certainty about the causes, natural course, and the relative merits of various treatment options. Hadn't President

Select Members of the Prostate Cancer Club
(identified by occupation or position for
which they are best known)

Current Members

Mason Adams	Actor
Ed Asner	Actor
Dusty Baker	Baseball manager, Chicago Cubs
Marion Barry	Mayor, Washington, DC
Harry Belafonte	Entertainer
Jim Berry	Cartoonist
Saxby Chambliss	U.S. senator, Georgia
Sean Connery	Actor
Len Dawson	NFL quarterback, Kansas City Chiefs
Robert De Niro	Actor
Bob Dole	U.S. senator, Kansas
Louis Farrakhan	Leader, Nation of Islam
Dan Fogelberg	Singer
George Foreman	Heavyweight boxer
Rudy Giuliani	Mayor, New York City
Robert Goulet	Actor
Merv Griffin	TV producer
Andy Grove	Businessman, cofounder and chairman of Intel
Jesse Helms	U.S. senator, North Carolina
Charlton Heston	Actor
Hamilton Jordan	White House chief of staff
George Karl	Coach, Denver Nuggets
Herb Kelleher	CEO, Southwest Airlines
John Kerry	U.S. senator, Massachusetts
Michael Korda	Editor in chief, Simon and Schuster
James Leach	Member of Congress, Iowa

Marv Levy	NFL coach, Buffalo Bills
Jerry Lewis	Actor
Nelson Mandela	President of South Africa
Michael Milken	Wall Street financier
Roger Moore	Actor
Robert Mueller	Director, FBI
Rupert Murdoch	Media owner
Stan Musial	Baseball player, Saint Louis Cardinals
Robert Novak	Journalist
Arnold Palmer	Professional golfer
Richard Petty	NASCAR driver
Sidney Poitier	Actor
Colin Powell	U.S. secretary of state
Pat Robertson	Televangelist
Norman Schwarzkopf	General, U.S. Army
Richard Shelby	U.S. senator, Alabama
Paul Stevens	U.S. Supreme Court justice
Ted Stevens	U.S. senator, Alaska
Joe Torre	Baseball manager, New York Yankees
Desmond Tutu	South African cleric
Andrew von Eschenbach	Director, National Cancer Institute
Andrew Young	Mayor, Atlanta

Past Members Who Died from Prostate Cancer,
with Age at Death

Don Ameche (85)	Actor
Wayne Calloway (62)	Chairman, Pepsico
Stokely Carmichael (Kwame Ture) (57)	Black activist
William Casey (68)	Director, CIA

Silvio Conte (69)	Member of Congress, Massachusetts
Gregory Corso (70)	Poet
Hume Cronyn (91)	Actor
Glenn Davis (80)	Heisman Trophy winner
Dean Gallo (59)	Member of Congress, New Jersey
John Gardner (89)	Founder, Common Cause
Ayatollah Khomeini (89)	Iranian cleric
Herbie Mann (73)	Jazz flutist
Spark Matsunaga (73)	U.S. senator, Hawaii
François Mitterand (79)	President of France
Marion Motley (79)	NFL player, Cleveland Browns
Jerry Orbach (69)	Actor
Joseph Papp (70)	Director, New York State Shakespeare Festival
Johnny Ramone (55)	Guitarist, founder of punk band
Bobby Riggs (77)	Tennis player
Steve Ross (65)	Chairman, Time Warner
Cornelius Ryan (54)	Writer
Telly Savalas (70)	Actor
William Shockley (79)	Physicist and Nobel laureate
Leo Szilard (66)	Scientist and writer
Pierre Trudeau (80)	Prime minister of Canada
Robert Penn Warren (84)	Writer
Willet Whitmore (78)	Expert on prostate cancer

Nixon declared war on cancer more than thirty years ago? What had my colleagues been doing all this time?

Second, the most useful information that was available was scattered in various professional papers, books, and websites. Much of it was out of date and contradictory, and some was factually wrong. Moreover, prominent urologists strongly disagreed with one another, publicly and not always politely, thus giving the appearance (ironic, given their profession) of an adolescent urinating contest. If

I, as a trained medical professional, was having trouble sorting it out and deciding what to do, what must nonprofessionals experience?

Finally, I was surprised to realize that I was the person who was expected to assess the treatment options and decide which one to select. I had grown up in an era when doctors usually made strong recommendations. Now, as noted by the *New York Times*, patients are awash in information, but "many find the job of being a modern patient, with its slog through medical uncertainty, to be lonely, frightening, and overwhelming."[4] Despite having an extremely supportive wife, an excellent internist and urologist, and many highly knowledgeable medical friends, I felt very much alone with my decision.

This book, then, is the book I wish had been available to me when I was diagnosed with prostate cancer. I hope it will lighten the load for other men who receive the same diagnosis.

2

How Serious Is Your Cancer?

S everal questions immediately came to mind on the day I was diagnosed with prostate cancer. How serious is it? Is it likely to kill me? If so, when? This chapter provides information you need to begin answering such questions. Those who wish to skip the more technical discussions will find a summary at the end of the chapter.

Prostate cancer *is* cancer. It affects the walnut-sized gland that sits beneath the bladder and contributes some of the fluid making up the semen; a detailed description of the prostate can be found in Appendix A. Prostate cancer should not be confused with benign prostatic hypertrophy (BPH), the other common—indeed, almost universal—prostate affliction of older men. For benign prostatic hypertrophy, the operant word is *benign*. It is an enlargement of the prostate that can cause symptoms such as frequency (having to urinate often), urgency (difficulty in holding your urine), a weak flow, and starting and stopping of the flow. Benign prostatic hypertrophy can be treated with medications or surgery. Sometimes, in the course of surgery for BPH, it is discovered incidentally that the enlarged prostate has cancer as well, but the two conditions are unrelated.

The following discussion assumes that the type of prostate cancer with which you have been diagnosed is an adenocarcinoma. More than 95 percent of all prostate cancers are of this type. The other 5 percent include small cell, squamous cell, sarcomas, and other rare types; all tend to be more aggressive and to have worse prognoses than adenocarcinomas.

The three most widely used indicators of severity in men with newly diagnosed prostate cancer are total prostate specific antigen (PSA) level; whether the cancer can be felt on digital rectal exam (often abbreviated as DRE) and an estimate of the cancer volume; and the appearance of the cancer cells obtained by biopsy (Gleason score). Other indicators of severity are not as widely used but may also be very useful; these are described below.

WHAT IS YOUR PSA?

Prostate specific antigen is a protein produced by cells in the prostate and, in very small amounts, by cells elsewhere in the body. PSA was discovered in 1979 and became widely used as a measure of prostate disease in the late 1980s. It is increased in most cases of prostate cancer, when the prostate is enlarged by benign prostatic hypertrophy and by inflammation of the prostate (prostatitis). Thus, PSA is a general measure of prostate pathology and is not specific for cancer.

Orgasm and ejaculation may increase PSA, and for this reason men are advised not to ejaculate for two days prior to having a PSA test. The level may also be elevated by massaging the prostate, as occurs during treatment for prostatitis, but should not be elevated by a normal digital rectal exam. There have been claims that vigorous bicycle and motorcycle riding may increase PSA by putting seat pressure on the prostate, but other studies do not agree. PSA is also partially determined by one's genes, so some men have higher PSA levels on a genetic basis alone. Conversely, PSA levels may be decreased in men who are obese and in men who are taking finasteride (Proscar) for BPH or finasteride (Propecia) to prevent baldness. Proscar and Propecia are the same drug, but Proscar contains a higher dose of finasteride (5 mg) than Propecia (1 mg). All these factors need to be taken into account when evaluating PSA level.

There is little agreement on the normal PSA level. However, there *is* agreement on one fact: PSA is a continuum, and the lower it is, the better off you are. Since most men's prostates increase in size as they age, what is considered to be a normal PSA level increases with age. A

What Is the Upper Limit of Normal PSA?

Many urologists now use age-corrected limits for normal PSA levels, recognizing that most men's prostates increase in size as they age, thereby increasing their PSA. The following have been recommended:

Ages 40–49:	Upper limit of 2.5
Ages 50–59:	Upper limit of 3.5
Ages 60–69:	Upper limit of 4.5
Ages 70 and above:	Upper limit of 6.5

Not everyone agrees with these figures; some urologists use lower levels.

---

level of 4 nanograms per milliliter of serum (hereafter written as PSA 4) has traditionally been regarded as the upper limit of normal, but increasingly urologists are using age-corrected upper limits (see box). The most important aspect of PSA, however, is the fact that it is a continuum, not positive or negative like a pregnancy test. Thus, there is virtually no difference between a PSA of 3.9 and 4.1, but a vast difference between 3.9 and 0.9.

Approximately 85 percent of men with prostate cancer have PSA levels higher than 4. However, that means that 15 percent of men with prostate cancer have PSA levels lower than 4. For example, General Schwarzkopf had a PSA of only 1.2 when he was diagnosed with prostate cancer. My own PSA level when I was diagnosed was 3.3, well within normal limits for a 66-year-old man. Well-described cases exist in which men with PSA levels of less than 1.0 have prostate cancers that have already spread to their lymph nodes and bones; fortunately, such cases are unusual.[1]

If your PSA is elevated, what are the chances that you have prostate cancer? If your PSA is between 4 and 10, the likelihood is about 25 percent. The majority of such elevations are caused by benign prostatic hypertrophy or by infections of the prostate. If your PSA is more than 10, the chances of your having cancer are over 50 percent. If your PSA is greater than 50, not only do you probably have cancer but it is likely to have already spread beyond the prostate. Charles Williams, in his book *That Black Men Might Live,* reveals that his PSA at the time of diagnosis was 172. In cases of metastatic disease in which the cancer has spread widely throughout the body, PSA levels can go higher than 1,000.

Because of widespread dissatisfaction with the use of total PSA as a marker for prostate cancer, attempts are being made to refine the test. One method is to separate the total PSA into its components, specifically the PSA fraction that is bound to other proteins in the blood and the fraction that is not bound (called *free PSA*). As a general rule, cancer cells make less free PSA than healthy prostate cells do. Therefore, the higher the fraction of free PSA in your blood, the greater the chances that you are free of cancer. One study reported that if the free PSA is more than 25 percent of the total PSA, the likelihood of having cancer is only 8 percent. At the other extreme, if the free PSA is less than 10 percent of the total PSA, the probability of having cancer is 56 percent. Michael Dorso, a physician who wrote about his own prostate cancer, knew he was in trouble when his free PSA report came back as 4 percent; he correctly noted that this was "not a good number!"[2] Free PSA measurements are more difficult to take than total PSA and thus are not available in some laboratories. This test is therefore underutilized.

Another promising use of PSA testing is to observe how rapidly the PSA is rising. This is called the *PSA velocity.* Any rise in PSA is a cause for concern, but a slow rise—for example, less than 0.75 in any given year—is less worrisome.[3] A PSA rise of more than 0.75 per year is more worrisome, and a rise of more than 2.0 in a year (for example, 1.3 to 3.4, or from 0.9 to 3.1) is very worrisome. Studies report that men with a PSA increase of more than 2.0 in the year prior to diagnosis of their cancer had a much higher death rate from their cancer, despite having treatment by surgery or radiation.[4]

The problem with PSA velocity, however, is that it is necessary to have had PSA measurements on an annual basis in order to use it. Most men do not undergo PSA testing that often, and many men do not have their PSA tested at all. *The potential importance of PSA velocity in predicting prostate cancer is a major reason why every man should have*

PSA Velocity Saves a Senator

An excellent example of the importance of PSA velocity is Senator John Kerry, who ran for President in 2004. In November 2002, during an annual checkup, Kerry had a PSA of 3.2, within the normal range for his age. However, Kerry's wife, Teresa Heinz Kerry, noted that his PSA had increased from 2.0 in December 1999 and 2.7 in February 2001 and urged him to have additional tests. In December 2002, a digital rectal exam was normal and his PSA was 3.4. Since Kerry's father had died of prostate cancer and because of the rise in his PSA, a biopsy was done, which found prostate cancer in five of the samples. Kerry subsequently underwent a radical prostatectomy and has had no recurrence of his cancer to date.

This case illustrates the importance of PSA velocity as a marker for prostate cancer. It also illustrates the benefit of having a wife who aggressively monitors her husband's health and, in this case, may have saved his life.

—adapted from L. K. Altman
New York Times, October 3, 2004

a baseline PSA test in his 40s and a regular PSA test from age 50 on (see Chapter 15). Since PSA testing varies somewhat between laboratories, it is advisable to have the testing performed by the same laboratory whenever possible.

IS YOUR CANCER PALPABLE?

The second indicator of severity that is widely used to evaluate men with newly diagnosed prostate cancer is whether the cancer can be felt on a digital rectal exam. The fact that 15 percent of prostate cancers have PSAs of less than 4 is sufficient reason for middle-aged and older men to have such an exam as part of their annual physical. The procedure, despite being undignified and mildly uncomfortable,

---

Getting a Second Opinion

Robert Hitchcock, in his book *Love, Sex, and PSA,* tells of a man who asked his urologist which finger he had used to examine the prostate during his digital rectal exam. The doctor replied that he had used his middle finger.

"Would you repeat the exam and use your index finger this time?" asked the patient.

"Why would you want me to do that?" replied the doctor.

"Because I would like to get a second opinion," said the man.

---

can discern many early-stage cancers that would otherwise go undetected until they became larger. The majority of prostate cancers begin in the posterior portion of the prostate gland, the area closest to the wall of the rectum. Thus, many small cancers can be perceived by an examining finger. The procedure has saved many lives, perhaps including my own.

When physicians doing rectal examinations feel something in the prostate that may be cancer, they try to estimate its size (volume) and also whether it occupies one or both sides of the gland. Such estimates are imprecise but nonetheless provide information regarding severity. *Prostate cancer volume* has been shown to be very important in predicting future course. In one study, men whose cancer involved 10 percent or more of the prostate had a 10 percent chance of recurrence, whereas men whose cancer involved 5 percent or less had a 5 percent rate of recurrence. In general, the larger the volume of the cancer, the greater the chance it has spread outside the prostate. Thomas Stamey, a prostate cancer researcher at Stanford University, has argued that prostate cancer volume and Gleason cell type (see below) are the two most important predictors of future course.[5] Cancer volume also correlates reasonably well with PSA level, with larger tumors producing higher PSAs.

Testing for Prostate Cancer

There's nothing like a battery of hospital tests to make you feel vulnerable, naked; as if your very life depends on them. As, indeed, it may. I had been living a quiet life, minding my business, not breaking the law. My time had felt free; which was what I had been used to; which I had always wanted; and still wanted. And now, suddenly, I was caught up in the full-fledged machinery of cancer; the machinery of what felt like a WAR. Tests. Questions. Debates. Crucial decisions. What was the enemy's local strength, position, logistics, tactics? What was his strategy? Above all, who would win?

—Charles Neider, *Adam's Burden*

Estimating the size of the prostate cancer is part of what is called staging the cancer. The Tumor, Node, Metastasis system, usually just abbreviated the TNM system, is most widely used. In this system, nonpalpable prostate tumors are labeled stage T1. Palpable tumors are labeled stage T2 and further divided as follows:

T2a. Palpable, but appears to involve less than half of one lobe
T2b. Palpable, and appears to involve more than half of one lobe but not both lobes
T2c. Palpable, and appears to involve both lobes

This numerical designation is included in the Partin tables, explained below, which are used to estimate the possible spread of the cancer. The main problem with this staging system is that it is imprecise. A somewhat better estimate of tumor volume can be obtained from the ultrasound examination done at the time of biopsy.

It is common for physicians to have patients with prostate cancer undergo bone scans after the initial diagnosis has been made. This procedure involves injecting a small amount of radioactive tracer into the bloodstream. The tracer is selectively absorbed by the bones, and the patient is examined by nuclear scanner; any spread of

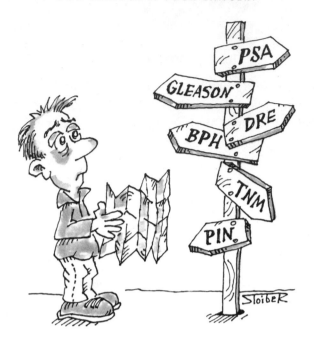

the cancer to the bones is visible as a "hot spot." Bone scans are negative for more than 95 percent of prostate cancer patients when first diagnosed, because in most cases the cancer has not spread or, if it has spread, it is too small to be detected on the scan. If it has spread, a different course of treatment is followed. I personally found the bone scan to be a benign procedure; lying on the scanning table in a semidarkened room seemed a fine opportunity for a short nap.

WHAT IS YOUR GLEASON SCORE?

The third indicator of severity used to evaluate men with newly di-agnosed prostate cancer is the *appearance* of the cells obtained by biopsy. Of the three indicators of severity, this is the most important.

In 1966 Donald Gleason, a pathologist at Johns Hopkins Univer-sity, proposed a classification of prostate cancer by appearance of the cells. He suggested grades 1 to 5, with 1 being the most benign and 5 the most malignant.

Grade 1. Cancer cells are well differentiated, with relatively normal ar-chitecture and clearly defined borders. They are arranged in a compact mass.

Grade 2. Cancer cells are still well differentiated, their arrangement is
more irregular, and occasional cell clusters are seen to invade
surrounding tissues.

Grade 3. Cancer cells are only moderately differentiated, their arrangement is quite irregular, and many cell groups are seen to be
invading surrounding tissue. This grade is the one most commonly seen in biopsy specimens.

Grade 4. Cancer cells are poorly differentiated, have distorted shapes,
and progressive invasion of surrounding tissues by cell clusters
is evident.

Grade 5. Cancer cells are grossly distorted, appear to melt together,
bear no resemblance to normal cells, and are no longer arranged in any formal clusters.

Cells that are intermediate between normal and grade 1 are commonly referred to as prostatic intraepithelial neoplasia, or PIN,
meaning that the prostate should be watched for possible problems.
Thought to be a precursor of future prostatic cancer, PIN is found in
about 5 percent of all prostate biopsies. When it is observed in an
otherwise normal prostate, most urologists recommend a rebiopsy
to make sure that an area of cancer has not been missed.

It is becoming increasingly clear that, from the point of view of
prognosis, the Gleason grading of cancer cells is not a continuum.
The majority of men with prostate cancer will be found to have grade
3 cancer cells on biopsy at the time of their initial diagnosis. The gaps
between grades 1 and 2 and grades 2 and 3 are not large, and individuals with all three cell types have very favorable prognoses. By contrast, the gap between grades 3 and 4 is large; men with grade 4 cells
have a significantly worse prognosis than men with grade 3 cells, and
the more grade 4 cells that are present, the worse the outlook. In one
study, men with grade 4 compared to grade 3 cells had an almost
threefold greater chance of having their cancer spread, and spread
more quickly. Men with grade 5 cells have an even worse prognosis,
but such men are fortunately few in number. One study reported
that the percentage of grade 4 and 5 cells in a tumor was the single
best predictor of recurrence of the prostate cancer.[6]

Classifying the cells in prostate cancer becomes more complicated, however, because almost all men with prostate cancer have
foci of cancer cells at several different sites in the prostate gland. In

Seeing Your Own Cancer

"Come take a look at this," the pathologist said. He and the urologist were peering through the separate eyepieces of a teaching microscope. I looked at the specimen, stained a delicate pink and blue, and followed as he showed me the nests of cancer cells infiltrating the normal architecture of the surrounding prostate gland. As I looked at the spread of these malignant interlopers, I felt dizzy.

"You guys go on without me," I said. "I'll meet you back in the room." The "room" was a gloomy examining room in the nearby urology clinic, adorned with pictures of diseased prostates. So I went and sat, still a bit unsteady, on the examining table. The prostate tissue was mine, the brightly colored product of a biopsy done 2 weeks earlier.

My colleagues at University Hospital assumed that I would want to join them in reviewing the biopsy. The biopsy was critical in selecting the best treatment option; the virulence, extent, and distribution of the cancer would determine whether I had a chance of being cured. But their fascinating intellectual exercise was my potential death sentence.

—Roger Rosenblatt, M.D., "Getting the News,"
Annals of Family Medicine

other words, prostate cancer, unlike most other cancers, is multifocal; therefore, almost every man affected can be said technically to have prostate cancers, not prostate cancer.

As he was devising his classification of cancer cells, Gleason was aware of this multifocal nature of prostate cancer. Accordingly, he proposed that the tumor should be classified twice: the first number grade would be for the cell type that was most frequent, and the second number grade would be for the cell type that was second most frequent. Thus was born the Gleason score, ranging from 2

(1+1) to 10 (5+5). Gleason scores of 2, 3, and 4 are rarely seen, because such cancers do not usually increase the PSA enough to call attention to themselves and are therefore not biopsied. A Gleason score of 6 (3+3) is the one most commonly reported in prostate biopsies; it means that only grade 3 cells were seen under the microscope.

A Gleason score of 7 is also common and presents problems for the Gleason scoring system. If the Gleason 7 score is a 3+4, it means that grade 4 cells constitute less than 50 percent; they could be as low as 5 percent and as high as 45 percent (gradings are done in increments of 5 percent). If, on the other hand, the Gleason 7 score is 4+3, then grade 4 cells are in the majority and could be as high as 95 percent. Grade 4 cells are significantly more malignant than grade 3 cells, so it is important to specify whether a Gleason 7 score is 3+4 or 4+3. A Gleason 7 (3+4) tumor, with few grade 4 cells, could have a relatively favorable prognosis close to that for a Gleason 6 cancer. Conversely, a Gleason 7 (4+3) tumor, with a high percentage of grade 4 cells, could have a relatively poor prognosis close to that for a Gleason 8 cancer. In one study of more than two thousand prostate cancers, those graded Gleason 7 (4+3) had a recurrence rate at seven and ten years double that for those graded Gleason 7 (3+4).[7]

Remember that the classification of cancer cell type in men who have been recently diagnosed with prostate cancer is based on the biopsy specimens. There is no guarantee that the biopsy material was obtained from representative sections of the multifocal tumor. In fact, when Gleason scores taken from biopsy specimens have been compared with Gleason scores taken from the complete cancer after it has been removed at surgery, it is found that the actual Gleason score is higher (for example, Gleason 6 on biopsy but Gleason 7 on surgical specimen) twice as often as it is found to be lower. This phenomenon is referred to as undergrading. Another problem in assessing your Gleason score is lack of agreement among pathologists; a 2005 study concluded that inter-rater agreement was only fair.[8]

In summary, three indicators of severity are commonly used to evaluate men with newly diagnosed prostate cancer. Although the total PSA is moderately helpful, it may be affected by other conditions. The percentage of free PSA and the rate of PSA rise (velocity) are probably more useful but are less widely available. The second indicator, whether the cancer is palpable on digital rectal exam and

Table 1. Percentage of Men with Cancers That Have Already Spread Outside the Prostate to the Seminal Vesicles and/or Lymph Nodes at the Time of Diagnosis (Abbreviated Version of Partin Tables)

| Gleason score | Cancer not felt on rectal exam (T1a) | Cancer appears to involve— | | |
		Less than half of one lobe (T2a)	More than half of one lobe (T2b)	Both lobes (T2c)
		PSA 0–2.5		
5–6	0%	1%	3%	2%
7 (3+4)	3	7	10	11
7 (4+3)	3	7	11	14
8–10	5	10	15	18
		PSA 2.6–4.0		
5–6	1	2	3	3
7 (3+4)	5	9	12	13
7 (4+3)	5	8	11	13
8–10	7	13	17	18
		PSA 4.1–6.0		
5–6	1	2	4	5
7 (3+4)	5	9	14	18
7 (4+3)	6	11	15	20
8–10	8	14	19	23
		PSA 6.1–10.0		
5–6	2	5	7	8
7 (3+4)	10	16	22	23
7 (4+3)	10	16	21	24
8–10	16	22	27	29
		PSA > 10.0		
5–6	6	10	16	19
7 (3+4)	18	30	39	46
7 (4+3)	21	31	40	48
8–10	28	36	46	53

NOTE: All numbers are approximations, within 95 percent confidence limits, and are based on specimens from 5,079 men who underwent surgery at Johns Hopkins Hospital between 1994 and 2000.

an estimate of the prostate cancer volume, depends in part on the skill of the examiner. The third indicator, the Gleason score, is probably the single best predictor of severity but has some limitations, especially for Gleason 7 cancers.

These three indicators of severity are commonly combined into tables to predict whether a given cancer has spread beyond the prostate. The tables were developed by Alan Partin at Johns Hopkins University, based on 5,079 surgical specimens examined between 1994 and 2000. They are usually referred to as Partin tables and are found in most books on prostate cancer. The abbreviated version shown in Table 1 allows a man to select the table covering his PSA score, then to select the stage of his cancer (whether it is palpable and, if so, its size), and finally to select the correct Gleason score. The result is a number that is the percentage chance that the cancer has spread beyond the prostate to involve the seminal vesicles and/or lymph nodes. Given the limitations of the data that go into the Partin tables, it is evident that the predictive value of these tables may or may not be accurate for any specific man.

These three indicators of severity are also used to divide prostate cancers into levels that predict the likelihood that the cancer will recur after treatment, as will be discussed in Chapter 11. The most widely used categories are those promoted by the National Comprehensive Cancer Network and the American Cancer Society:

Low chance of recurrence
- Not palpable on rectal exam (T1) or, if palpable, occupies less than half of one lobe (T2a); and
- Gleason score 6 or lower; and
- PSA below 10.

Intermediate chance of recurrence
- Occupies both halves of one lobe (T2b) or both lobes (T2c); or
- Gleason score 7; or
- PSA 10–20.

High chance of recurrence
- Tumor has spread beyond prostate capsule; or
- Gleason score 8–10; or
- PSA above 20.

Very high chance of recurrence
- Tumor has spread to seminal vesicles, lymph nodes, or more distantly to bones or other organs.

ADDITIONAL PREDICTORS OF SEVERITY

It would be helpful if we had more accurate indicators of severity for men with newly diagnosed prostate cancers. Our treatment decisions, and even whether to pursue treatment at all, are currently based on inadequate data. If we were better able to predict which cancers are likely to remain quiescent and which are likely to progress, many men would not have to undergo treatment and could thereby avoid complications such as incontinence and impotence. The fact that we do not have valid indicators of severity results from the failure of prostate cancer research (see Chapter 14).

Additional predictors of severity are available from prostate biopsies but are underutilized. These include information on the number of specimens (cores) positive for cancer, the percentage of each positive core occupied by cancer, and the percentage of Gleason grade 4 or 5 cells in each core. For example, my own biopsy included 9 probes, 5 on the right side (where the cancer had been felt) and 4 on the left side. On the right, 3 of the 5 had cancer, and on the left 0 of 4 did. Thus, overall, 3 of 9 were positive.

Several studies have reported that the percentage of biopsy probes that are positive for cancer is a better predictor of recurrence than the PSA level. In a large study of 1,149 prostate cancer biopsies, only 1 core was positive for cancer in 47 percent of cases; 2 in 24 percent; 3 in 18 percent; and 4 or more in 11 percent. One study focused specifically on Gleason 7 cancers and reported that when one third or fewer cores were positive for cancer, chances of cancer recurrence after surgery were significantly lower than if one half or more cores were positive. Another study reported that the percentage of biopsy cores positive for cancer was the best predictor of cancer recurrence for men undergoing beam radiation treatment.[9]

Biopsy reports also usually include information on what percentage of each positive core is occupied by cancer cells. In two of my positive cores, cancer involved 20 percent of the specimen; in the third core, it involved 5 percent. Furthermore, Gleason grade 4 cells occupied 40 percent of the cancer in one core, 20 percent in another core, and there were no grade 4 cells in the third core. Studies suggest that the percentage of cancer in the positive cores and the percentage of the cancer that is Gleason grade 4 and 5 cells are both predictive of outcome. One study reported that if cancer in any positive core occupies more than 50 percent of the core, the chances of cancer recurrence is 15 percent higher at five years and 30 percent higher at ten years than if the cancer occupies less than 50 percent of the core.[10] And for Gleason 7 cancers, the greater the percentage of grade 4 cells in the positive cores, the more serious the cancer.

Attempts to identify additional and more accurate indicators of severity in newly diagnosed prostate cancers continue. Such indicators include specific proteins in the blood and urine, as well as measurement of genes that have become activated; these will be discussed in Chapter 15. Advances in this research area could profoundly affect how we treat prostate cancer.

In summary, the best predictors of having prostate cancer and of the severity of such cancers are the following:

- PSA level: below 4 is favorable; 4–10, you have a 25 percent chance of having cancer; 10–20, you have a 50 percent chance of having cancer; the higher the level over 20, the greater the chance of your having cancer and the more serious the cancer is likely to be.
- Free PSA: the lower the free PSA as a percentage of total PSA, the more likely it is that you have cancer; over 25 percent is a good sign; under 10 percent is not a favorable sign.
- PSA velocity: the faster the PSA rises, the more likely it is that you have cancer; a very rapid increase in PSA suggests a rapidly growing cancer. In order for this measure to be useful, you must have had multiple PSA measurements over time.
- If the cancer is large enough to be felt on digital rectal exam, that is not a favorable sign.
- The larger the size (volume) of the cancer, the more serious it is likely to be.
- If cancer is felt in only one-half of one lobe of the prostate, that is good. If it is felt in both halves of one lobe, the outlook is not quite so favorable. If it is felt in both halves (both lobes) of the prostate, that is less favorable.

- A Gleason score (the combination of two numbers) of 5 or less is very good. A score of 6 is still good. A score of 7 (3+4) or 7 (4+3) is not as good, but the seriousness depends on the percentage of grade 4 cells present. A score of 8 or more is not favorable.
- Each biopsy consists of a number of cores. The fewer cores positive for cancer, the better your chances of having a curable cancer.
- Each biopsy core that has cancer is assessed for the percentage of the total core that is cancerous. If the core that has the most cancer has less than 50 percent, that is good.
- Any sign of spread of cancer outside the prostate is definitely not favorable.

CHAPTER

3

Surgical Treatment

The surgical removal of prostate cancer has for many years been the most common treatment of the disease. It has been controversial, with proponents arguing that surgery is the only real hope for permanently curing the cancer, and opponents claiming that the main effect of surgery is to produce incontinence and impotence without any clear evidence, compared to other forms of treatment, that it actually lengthens men's lives.

The surgical removal of enlarged prostates, both those caused by benign prostatic hypertrophy and those resulting from cancer, has a long history. Until the middle of the twentieth century, the operation was carried out through an incision in the perineum, the area between the back of the scrotum and the anus. During the past half-century it has become more popular to surgically remove cancerous prostates through an abdominal incision, an operation referred to as a radical retropubic prostatectomy. The term *radical* is used because lymph nodes and other tissues surrounding the prostate are routinely removed by the surgeon as well as the prostate itself. Because of its location, surgical removal of the prostate is technically a difficult operation, although in the skilled hands of an experienced urologist it has become fairly routine.

WHO ARE GOOD CANDIDATES?

The best candidates for surgery are younger men whose cancer is in a relatively early stage. An example would be a man in his fifties with a cancer detected by PSA, not yet palpable on rectal exam, and a Gleason score of 5 or 6. One study reported that "men 50 years old or younger had significantly lower recurrence rates than did older men" and that recurrence rates increased with the age of the patient at the time of surgery.[1]

Younger men with prostate cancer are much more likely to be offered, and to select, surgical treatment. In a Canadian study, 59 percent of men younger than 60 years of age chose surgery, compared to only 6 percent who chose radiation. By contrast, for men aged 60 to 69, the percentage who chose surgery and radiation was the same.[2] The fact that younger men with prostate cancer are more likely to choose surgery is problematic insofar as these are the men for whom impotence, a common side effect of surgery, is apt to be the most keenly felt; but it is also true that younger men will more probably recover sexual function following surgery.

Some urologists have argued that surgery is most likely to be effective for men whose cancer is at an intermediate stage of development—likely to spread but having not yet done so. Examples of such cases are palpable tumors with a Gleason score of 6 and a PSA level of 10 to 20; Gleason 7 (3+4) tumors; and possibly Gleason 7 (4+3) tumors in which grade 4 cells occupy the majority but not most of the tumor. Surgical removal in such cases, it is argued, can truly be lifesaving.

Surgical removal of the prostate is a major operation that usually takes two to three hours but may take longer; therefore, men with other serious diseases are not considered to be appropriate candidates. One study reported that men with heart disease, disease of their arteries, chronic lung disease, or severe kidney disease all had an elevated death rate following prostate cancer surgery; but such men are poor candidates for any type of major surgery. Further, as will be discussed in Chapter 8, the principal survival advantages of surgical treatment for prostate cancer, compared to radiation, may not become evident until fifteen years or more after surgery. Thus, candidates for surgery should have a remaining life expectancy of at

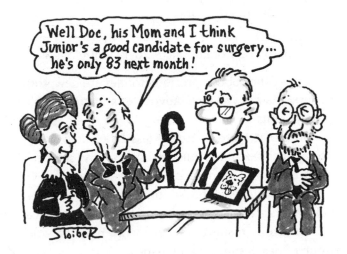

least fifteen more years. In the Canadian study cited above, only 3 percent of men aged 70 to 79 chose surgical treatment. When Johns Hopkins University urologist Patrick Walsh was asked whether he would ever consider surgical treatment for a man with prostate cancer who was 80 years old, he replied: "Only if he were brought in by his parents."[3]

Most surgeons restrict candidates for surgery to those in whom the cancer is thought to be confined to the prostate. If the cancer has already spread, it is reasoned, surgical removal will accomplish nothing. Not all surgeons agree, however, and some remove the prostate in cases in which the cancer is known to have spread, under the theory that removal will slow additional spread and make hormone and/or radiation treatments more effective.

THE PROCEDURE

A prostatectomy necessitates an average hospital stay of two days and a minimum of three weeks' recuperation. It can be carried out under general anesthesia or with a local block (spinal or epidural) in which the patient is awake but feels nothing. When a local block is used, the patient is also given sedation and usually sleeps through the operation. Some surgeons and anesthesiologists have strong preferences regarding which form of anesthesia to use, whereas others let the patient decide.

Is Laparoscopic or Robotic Surgery Right for You?

Laparoscopic and robotic prostatectomies are new; thus few follow-up data are available. Advocates and critics make the following points:

- All agree that there is usually less blood loss, less pain, shorter hospitalization, quicker recovery, and smaller scars.
- Some claim the camera provides better vision. Others claim the surgeons cannot see the whole field and, because their fingers are not used in the operative field, they cannot feel cancerous tissue that is palpable but not visible in lymph nodes or surrounding tissues.
- Some claim the computerized system permits a more precise dissection of the nerves next to the prostate and thus improves the chances of retaining erections. Others doubt this. There is as yet no long-term follow-up to ascertain the facts.
- Some claim that preliminary studies with these methods have reported a higher rate of positive margins, meaning that some cancer may have been left behind. Others say this occurs only with inexperienced surgeons.
- All agree that the cost of surgery using the robotic system is extremely high and may not be fully covered by medical insurance.
- All agree that laparoscopic and robotic surgery is technically very demanding and difficult to learn. Men selecting this option should choose a surgeon who has performed at least thirty such surgeries. (The question is, on whom should those thirty surgeries be done?)

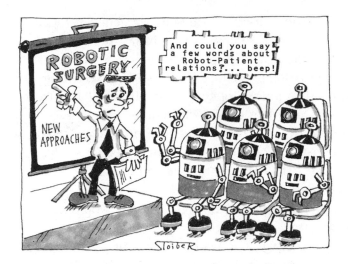

In most cases a vertical, abdominal incision is made, stretching from the umbilicus to just above the penis; this is the retropubic prostatectomy. A perineal approach, in which a small horizontal incision is made between the back of the scrotum and the anus, is also possible; it can be useful for men who are obese, but may present problems if the tumor is very large. A perineal prostatectomy is much less commonly performed now than it was in the past.

In the last decade, laparoscopic prostatectomies have been introduced in which the procedure is carried out with long instruments through multiple small abdominal incisions. This surgery is technically very demanding and is presently performed in only a few centers, but it is rapidly becoming more widely available. Proponents claim that it produces less blood loss, less postoperative pain, and quicker recovery. All the same, laparoscopic prostatectomies have been described by one surgeon as being like "backing a tractor trailer around a curve by looking through the rearview mirror."[4]

A variant of laparoscopic surgery is surgery performed by a robot, which the surgeon guides by using a computer. The surgeon may be seated several feet from the patient, or theoretically could even operate while sitting in the next room. Three computer-controlled robotic arms do the actual surgery: one holds a video camera, and the other two hold tiny tools for cutting, suturing, and so on. The robotic system most widely used is the da Vinci system developed by the U.S. military; the robot costs approximately $1.2 million.

Surgical removal of the prostate can be carried out in many cases via a nerve-sparing procedure. This approach, developed in 1982 by Patrick Walsh at Johns Hopkins University and Pieter Donker in the Netherlands, involves careful dissection of the nerves to the penis that run immediately next to the prostate gland. When the nerves are preserved, the chances of retaining erections after surgery are increased. In 10 to 20 percent of prostate cancer cases, it is not possible to preserve one or both nerves, because the cancer is immediately adjacent to them, and preserving the nerves would risk leaving cancer cells behind.

Most surgeons like to wait at least four weeks after the biopsy before doing surgery; this delay gives the rectal wall a chance to heal and decreases the likelihood of injuring the wall as the prostate is removed. In addition, it provides the man who has decided on surgery an opportunity to take care of necessary tasks.

All blood-thinning medications including warfarin (Coumadin), aspirin, and aspirin-containing over-the-counter medications should be stopped at least ten days prior to surgery. Many surgeons ask patients to donate two units of blood for use during surgery, since the average blood loss is between one and one and a half units. Some surgeons ask men to take iron pills to build up their blood before the surgery. Men should also discuss anesthesia with the surgeon and/or anesthesiologist.

One of the things I personally found helpful before surgery was planning how I would spend my "post-op" recuperation period. I went to a video store and made a list of old movies I wanted to see. My wife recommended comedies, but I selected mostly the tragedies of Ingmar Bergman; they seemed more in keeping with the occasion. I also did all the yard work I could, knowing that it would be depressing to sit on the porch during my recovery and look at the jobs not done.

Another presurgical task I found helpful was to visualize myself entering the hospital, taking off my clothes, putting on a surgical gown (it hardly warrants such a designation), and being wheeled into the operating room. It was also helpful to have visited the hospital for my presurgical procedures. Although I am a physician, my

Things to Do Prior to Surgery

- Check your insurance coverage.
- Draw up and sign a living will if you do not already have one.
- If you are employed, check your sick-leave policy and arrange coverage of your tasks for at least three weeks following the surgery.
- Stop warfarin (Coumadin), aspirin, and all medications containing aspirin (Anacin, Bufferin, and the like) at least ten days prior to surgery.
- Donate two units of blood for use during your surgery, and take iron pills if your surgeon recommends it.
- Discuss anesthesia options with your surgeon and/or an anesthesiologist.
- Plan for your initial weeks of recuperation.
- If you live alone, make arrangements to have someone stay with you for the first week after surgery.
- Visualize yourself going to the hospital and into surgery. The image will decrease your anxiety when you actually do so.

relationship with surgeons and hospitals was a distant one on the best of days. My only personal surgical experiences were having had my tonsils removed as a child under ether anesthesia (which I clearly recall produced a feeling of suffocation), and the surgical repair of a fracture under local nerve block anesthesia that did not really block the nerve. Thus, I could identify with General Schwarzkopf who, in discussing his own lack of enthusiasm for surgery, said, "I go into a kung-fu attack position when I go through the door of a hospital."[5] Men who have previously undergone other major surgery are likely to have an easier time with prostate cancer surgery than those who have not.

On the day prior to surgery, you are restricted to a clear liquid diet, and the night before, you are instructed to give yourself a Fleet

enema. Entering the hospital for the surgery proved to be less onerous than I had anticipated, thanks to having practiced visualizing
it and to the support of my wife. Nevertheless, the temptation remained to suddenly declare that watchful waiting was the better
treatment—and bolt. I was scheduled as the first case of the day, an
arrangement I recommend so that you do not have to lie around
waiting. My surgeon greeted me; I briefly contemplated asking him
to replace my degenerating hip while he was working on my prostate, since it was anatomically close by. However, I decided that although I was certain about his surgical skills, I was *un*certain about
his sense of humor. In the operating room, I surveyed the operating
room staff, reassured myself that they appeared alert, then suddenly
was asleep.

I vaguely recall awakening in the recovery room and being asked
questions. I do not recall feeling much pain, but I have a high pain
threshold, so I may not be an accurate gauge. I apparently answered
questions correctly, because I was wheeled to my room and my waiting spouse. I considered rolling my eyes up in my head and letting
my tongue hang out the side of my mouth as a novel greeting but
calculated—correctly, I was later told—that even a strong marriage
might not withstand such a shock.

Despite being groggy from the anesthesia, I felt it necessary to
reconnoiter my anatomy. I had an intravenous tube in one arm, and
my legs were enveloped in pneumatic stockings that effectively tied
my legs to the bottom of the bed. Every minute or so, the mecha-
nized stockings slowly massaged my legs, a process described by one
man as "coiling upwards, squeezing you from ankle to thigh like two
pet boas in estrus."[6] The stockings decrease the probability of blood
clots in your legs. My lower abdomen was covered with a large dressing, and an adjacent smaller dressing covered the opening for the
surgical drain. A urinary catheter exited my penis and ran to a bag
attached to the bed. My penis and the surrounding tissues were partially black-and-blue. I was beginning to understand the meaning of
the "major" in major surgery.

And then, with a shock, I noticed: my penis looked a little
shorter! I recalled a passage in *Dr. Patrick Walsh's Guide to Surviving
Prostate Cancer*:

Note that the gap between the bladder and urethra—where the prostate used to be—is now filled by the bladder. Some men worry that the penis will be shortened—that the surgeon will pull it up to meet the bladder. This doesn't happen; instead the bladder is mobile, and can easily be pulled down to meet the urethra.[7]

The book's reassurance notwithstanding, the visual evidence was compelling. Most men pay close attention to such details. My initial reaction was a mix of incredulity and amusement, and I wondered how many *other* things that I had read about prostate surgery were mistaken.

A few weeks later, I surveyed the medical literature regarding this phenomenon. Two studies reported that, when measured before prostate surgery and three months later, two thirds of men showed a decrease in penile length. In the majority of cases, the decrease was minimal, but in some men it was 15 percent or more. One man wrote that his genitals "had shrunk and receded into [his] body to such an extent that they surely would have been safe from Lorena Bobbitt."[8]

Over time, the decrease in penile length becomes less noticeable and does not seem to affect penile function. Some urologists have attributed the shortening to disuse or fibrosis of the penis, but this is obviously not the case, since the shortening is visible immediately post-op. A more likely explanation is that it is a reaction to the inevitable small-nerve damage during surgery. The bottom line is that nobody seems to know the cause, but denying that the decrease may occur is not helpful when the facts are otherwise.

On the day of surgery, I received intravenous ketoralac (Toradol) for pain and did not feel much discomfort. Toradol is a strong, non-steroidal anti-inflammatory drug that should not be taken for more than five days because of its propensity for causing peptic ulcers or gastrointestinal bleeding. It can also generate nausea or diarrhea. It made me drowsy, so I slept much of the day and woke up at two in the morning. Fortunately, I had brought headphones and CDs with me and spent most of the night listening to classical music, pleased that I had survived the ordeal. My private room was well worth the extra expense and allowed my wife to spend the night there as well.

The following morning, twenty-four hours after surgery, one of the urologists checked me and asked if I wanted to go home. This seemed extraordinary, but is typical of hospital stays in the era of managed care. I allowed that I thought I would stay for another day; if I had been living alone, I would have stayed longer. Nevertheless, because of the risk of hospital-acquired infections, hospitals are dangerous places to spend time unnecessarily and no one should stay longer than is absolutely essential. I spent the day walking the hall with my catheter bag, accompanied by other prostatectomy patients. In *My Prostate and Me,* William Martin describes a similar scene as "the few, the humiliated, the Urine Corps" and adds: "One look at my new peer group moved me to suggest that it might be best if would-be visitors just sent a note or called. Men look better in power suits."[9]

By day 2 after surgery, I was ready to go home but had two urgent questions for my urologist: What did the pathology report say about whether my cancer was confined to the prostate, and had he saved one or both nerves? The second question was quickly answered: one (as I had suspected would be the case from the size and position of the cancer). To answer the first question, my urologist went to the pathology department himself and reviewed the slides with the pathologist. The cancer had penetrated the capsule but had not gone through it and had a "negative margin," meaning that the cancer appeared to have been confined to the tissue removed at surgery. There was also no spread to the seminal vesicles or lymph nodes. This was all positive news.

The first two weeks of recuperation were surprisingly pleasant. My wife and I read, took short walks, and watched movies each afternoon before having a drink. I was surprised at how easily I became fatigued and I took a nap each day. I also listened to a CD series on the history of science and sat in the sun. I was fortunate to have only occasional pain, such as when I sneezed and thereby increased the abdominal pressure; I used no pain medication after leaving the hospital. Some nurses recommend a firm "laugh pillow" to hold against your abdomen when you laugh, sneeze, or cough. It is also important to not become constipated, which can be caused by pain medications such as codeine, by iron pills, and by inactivity; constipation can be avoided by taking laxatives. (I elected not to take iron pills

Of Dogs and Catheters

Geoff Barnard of Flagstaff, Arizona, wrote the following account of his adventures with a catheter after having a radical prostatectomy for prostate cancer:

> Several nights ago here at home I woke up to our smoke alarm going off. That scared the dog, Copper, who dove under the bed and in so doing got my catheter tube wrapped around her neck. So imagine my fun, grabbing the tube with a forty-five-pound terrified dog pulling in the other direction, screaming to Diane to hold the dog and get it unwrapped, with the smoke alarm going off all the while. It will be hard to top that with an encore!

after surgery, as had been recommended to build up my blood count, in order to avoid possible constipation.)

My main post-op problem was the catheter, which rubbed my penis and made it sore. Anchoring the catheter tube with safety pins to my pant leg seemed to help. Others have recommended putting K-Y jelly or antibiotic ointment around the opening of the penis to minimize irritation. You are given a small catheter bag that straps to your leg to use during the day; it allows you to take walks and move about freely. At night, you hook a large catheter bag to the side of the bed. Bert Gottlieb, writing of his experience in *The Men's Club,* said that he christened his small catheter bag "Rover," because it followed him everywhere.[10]

My recuperative turning point came with the removal of the catheter and suture clips at ten days; contrary to what I had been told, the first did not hurt, but the second did, briefly. Some surgeons leave the catheter in for up to three weeks. Its removal meant that I was on my own to either recover urinary continence or not. My urologist had advised me to bring to the hospital what is essentially an adult diaper (see Chapter 10) to wear home, but even as I did so,

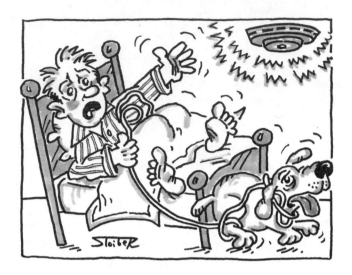

I felt as if I was getting well. I resumed driving, which also made me feel better.

Recovering urinary function after prostate surgery is an interesting experience. It is as if you have been living in an old house for many years and are familiar with the sounds of its plumbing. You know when someone downstairs flushes the toilet and when somebody upstairs is taking a shower. When your house is completely renovated with new plumbing, all the old familiar cues are gone and you have to learn new ones. I was fortunate that my external sphincter was up to the task. Continence returned quickly. I discarded the adult diaper the first day and thereafter used pads of varying sizes for three weeks. After that, I needed nothing, and in fact had less dribbling than I had had prior to surgery. Some men are not so fortunate; Michael Korda's account in *Man to Man* describes the problems that occur when continence does not return quickly.

After three weeks I returned to work but restricted my hours. Some men recover more slowly and take more time off. My strength gradually returned. At six weeks post-op, at which time my urologist said I could resume normal activities, my wife and I went on a planned vacation to Newfoundland to do some gentle sea kayaking. It was not until approximately three months after surgery, however, that I felt that my full strength had returned.

COMPLICATIONS

Surgical removal of the prostate carries the same risk of complications as does all major surgery. These include infection, post-op bleeding, and the ultimate complication, death. The death rate in the first thirty days following prostatectomy, according to a 2005 Canadian study, is less than 2 in 1,000 for men under age 60, and 6 in 1,000 for men 60 to 79.[11] The most important cause of death is thrombosis (clots) of the veins in the legs, which often causes tenderness in the calf or leg swelling; when clots break free, they may travel to the lungs and heart as emboli and cause shortness of breath, chest pain, and sometimes sudden death. The best prevention is to get patients up and walking soon after surgery and to maintain regular walking and leg exercises for several weeks.

While the catheter is in place, a small number of men have bladder spasms, which are painful contractions of the bladder as it tries to expel the catheter. Korda describes these in *Man to Man;* in most cases, the spasms can be alleviated with medication. Some men develop a narrowing of the urethra where it is surgically attached to the bladder, and thus a narrowing of the urinary stream. Severe cases of this bladder neck obstruction require surgical dilation, which can be done as an outpatient procedure.

The three most common complications of all treatments for prostate cancer are urinary incontinence, impotence, and bowel dysfunction. Incontinence rates after surgical removal of the prostate vary widely and are a source of spirited debate among urologists. Some of the differences are due to variable levels of skill among surgeons. Some result from different definitions of incontinence; for example, some researchers use "frequent leakage" as a definition, whereas others use "wears pads." One man's definitions of "frequent" and "leakage" may differ substantially from another man's definitions, and one man may wear a pad for occasional, minimal leakage while another may not wear one despite having copious leakage.

Incontinence rates also vary depending on whether the physician is making the assessment or whether the information comes from questionnaire self-reports from the patients. As one publication noted: "Treating physicians in these studies report complication rates that are generally low, but may be inaccurate because patients may minimize complication of treatment to their doctors, who in turn may subconsciously discount patient reports of symptoms."[12]

Finally, incontinence rates vary depending on the patient group being followed, with young men with low-grade tumors having the fewest problems.

The lowest rates of urinary incontinence following prostate surgery have been claimed by the Johns Hopkins University group who, for a small group of fifty-nine patients, reported that only 7 percent were wearing pads eighteen months after surgery. This was a highly select group of patients, however, with an average age of 57 and early stage tumors (88 percent Gleason 6 or less; 85 percent PSA less than 10). A much more representative group of patients is the 1,291 men from six different areas in the United States surveyed by the Prostate Cancer Outcomes Study. At two years following prostate surgery, 22 percent were wearing pads. This group was substantially older (72 percent age 60 and older) and had had more advanced cancers (only 56 percent Gleason 6 or less) than the Johns Hopkins cohort. Other studies that have assessed urinary continence in men following prostate surgery have reported results closer to those of the Prostate Cancer Outcomes Study.[13]

It thus appears that some degree of urinary incontinence is a common complication following prostatectomy. Approximately 20 percent of men use pads for at least occasional leakage, although studies suggest that the incontinence is severe in fewer than 10 percent of men. There is also consensus that the incontinence is most likely to occur in the early months after surgery and usually improves over time.

Impotence is a common complication of prostate surgery and, like incontinence, its assessment is made more difficult by varying definitions and the selection of patients. Should impotence be defined as inability to have an erection at all? An erection firm enough to have intercourse? With or without pharmacological help?

When we review the varied and contradictory studies on impotence that have been published, three findings stand out. First, the younger a man is at the time of surgery, the better are his chances of regaining potency. Second, a man who had satisfactory sexual function prior to surgery is much more likely to have a favorable outcome after surgery. Third, erectile function can return very slowly follow-ing surgery; according to one review, it "continues to improve after radical prostatectomy up to at least 2 years after treatment."[14] This slow rate is consistent with what is known about nerve regeneration after nerves have been traumatized, even when they have not been severed.

That being said, let me emphasize that, in the words of one re-search group, "few men undergoing radical prostatectomy even-tually achieve the preoperative level of erectile function."[15] Impo-tence is a major complication—for most men, *the* major complication —of prostate surgery. The reported rates of impotence vary widely, however, and are hotly disputed.

At one end of the spectrum is the Johns Hopkins University study described above, which included a small, select sample of young men with early-stage prostate cancer. Walsh and his col-leagues claimed that the impotence rate among these men was 62 percent at three months post-op; 46 percent at six months; 27 per-cent at twelve months; and 14 percent at eighteen months. Else-where, Walsh has claimed that, if both nerves are preserved during surgery, the rate of impotence should be no higher than 20 percent for men in their forties and fifties, and no higher than 40 percent for men in their sixties.[16]

Other researchers have claimed that the Johns Hopkins numbers represent select patients and are unrealistically optimistic. The large and more representative Prostate Cancer Outcomes Study reported an overall rate of impotency of 60 percent eighteen months after surgery; the rate for men who had had both nerves preserved was 56 percent, only slightly better than the overall rate. Other studies have reported even higher rates of impotence, including rates of 75 per-cent and 80 percent at twelve months post-op.[17] Most of these stud-ies defined men as potent if they were able to achieve an erection sufficient for intercourse, with or without the assistance of sildenafil (Viagra) or other oral medication.

It is clear that nerve-sparing surgery is effective in decreasing the rate of postsurgical impotence. Although little advantage was reported by the Prostate Cancer Outcomes Study, other studies have disagreed. A large study of 1,014 men aged 60 to 70 reported that 92 percent of the men were impotent when neither nerve was preserved during surgical removal of the prostate, but that only 66 percent were impotent when one or both nerves were preserved. The authors concluded: "Most of the studies using patient-report, validated, questionnaire methodology have corroborated that nerve-sparing technique is associated with better sexual . . . recovery after radical prostatectomy than the non-nerve sparing technique."[18] Because of the size of the cancer, it is sometimes not possible to spare both nerves.

In summary, impotence is a serious problem for men following prostate surgery. For men in their 60s in whom one or both nerves have been preserved, the impotence rate ranges between 40 and 80 percent. Younger men fare somewhat better, especially those who had satisfactory presurgical sexual function. Men in whom both nerves have been cut during surgery will almost all be impotent.

The third major complication of prostate cancer treatment is disturbance in bowel function, such as crampy pain, diarrhea, and bowel urgency. For individuals who elect surgery, this is usually not a significant problem. A large study of 1,296 men who had surgical treatment for prostate cancer reported minor bowel symptoms in some men and found that "this is short-lived, and during the first 3 months after surgery bowel function improves significantly" and essentially returns to normal.[19]

OUTCOME

Many men believe that if their prostate cancer is removed surgically and if there are no signs that the cancer has spread, then they are cured. This belief has been fostered by enthusiasts for prostate cancer surgery and by media presentations. The author of a 1996 *Time* magazine article about prostate cancer claimed that surgical treatment is "the only one that can virtually guarantee a cure—if the cancer has not metastasized. . . . If the cancer has not spread beyond the prostate wall and the gland is removed, the cancer is gone. Period."[20]

Unfortunately, that is not always true. Recurrence of prostate cancer following surgery is not a rare event. Two factors strongly influence the chance of recurrence: the age of the man and the stage of the cancer. The younger the man is at the time of surgery, the better his chances that the cancer will be curable. In one study of more than three thousand patients, the chances of cancer recurrence ten years after surgery were 24 percent in men 41 to 50; 29 percent in men aged 51 to 60; 34 percent in men 61 to 70; and 37 percent in men over 70. In another study in which all the men had PSAs between 4 and 6, only 13 percent of men aged 40 to 50 were considered to be not cured (defined by the pathological characteristics of the cancer), compared to 19 percent of men 51 to 60 and 26 percent of men 61 to 73. In this study, the age of the man was a better predictor of outcome than was the presurgical PSA level.[21]

The stage of prostate cancer is determined by the Gleason score and other pathological features, as described in Chapter 2. In one study that compared men who all had nonpalpable tumors, those who had a Gleason score of 6 or less and a PSA of 10 or less had only a 4 percent chance of cancer recurrence at ten years; by contrast, those who had a Gleason score of 7 or more and a PSA over 10 had a 27 percent chance of cancer recurrence. In another study of men followed for more than twenty years after surgery, those whose cancer was confined to the prostate at the time of surgery had a 27 percent rate of recurrence; those whose cancer was not so confined had an 83 percent rate of recurrence.[22]

An important question in research on the outcome of prostate cancer treatment is how the outcome is measured. Following surgery, the PSA level should drop to virtually zero, since the prostate has been removed and the amount of PSA made by other tissues is negligible. For this reason, it is common practice among urologists to assume that any PSA level of 0.2 or higher means that some cancer cells spread beyond the prostate at the time of surgery and that the cancer has recurred. Some urologists use a PSA of 0.4 or higher rather than 0.2 as an indication of recurrence. As will be discussed in Chapter 11, recurrence measured by PSA alone does not necessarily mean that the cancer will progress.

Another measure of cancer recurrence is that it has spread (metastasized) to the lymph nodes, bones, or other organs. Such cancers usually continue to spread and eventually lead to death if the man does not die from another cause. The ultimate measure of treatment for prostate cancer is how often the cancer kills. Another way to look at outcome is to assess whether treatment lengthens a patient's life beyond what he would have lived naturally or would have lived with

Table 2. Follow-up Studies of Recurrence Rates and Prostate Cancer Deaths
Following Surgery for Prostate Cancer

	Houston: Baylor	St. Louis: Washington University	Rochester, Minn.: Mayo Clinic	Baltimore: Johns Hopkins
Number of men:	1,000	3,478	3,170	2,404
Average age:	63	61	66	58
Years of surgery:	1983–1998	1983–2003	1966–1991	1982–1999
Average follow-up:	4.4 years	5.4 years	5.0 years	6.3 years
% recurrence measured by PSA				
10 years:	25	32	48	26
15 years:			60	34
% metastases				
10 years:	16	NA	18	10
15 years:			24	18
% dead because of prostate cancer				
10 years:	2	3	10	6
15 years:			18	10

SOURCE: G. W. Hull, F. Rabbani, F. Abbas, et al., Cancer control with radical prostatectomy alone in 1,000 consecutive patients, *Journal of Urology* 67 (2002): 528–534; K. A. Roehl, M. Han, C. G. Ramos, et al., Cancer progression and survival rates, *Journal of Urology* 172 (2004): 910–914; H. Zincke, J. E. Oesterling, M. L. Blute, et al., Long-term (15 years) results after radical prostatectomy for clinically localized (stage T2c or lower) prostate cancer, *Journal of Urology* 152 (1994): 1850–57; M. Han, A. W. Partin, C. R. Pound, et al., Long-term biochemical disease-free and cancer-specific survival following anatomic radical retropubic prostatectomy, *Urologic Clinics of North America* 28 (2001): 555–565.

prostate cancer if he had not been treated at all; both of these factors are discussed in Chapter 8.

Four large studies assessed the recurrence rates and cancer-related death rates following surgery for prostate cancer. Because the studies included men of different ages and with different stages of cancer and also used different outcome measures, it is difficult to compare them. The studies were carried out at Baylor College of Medicine in Houston, Washington University School of Medicine in St. Louis, the Mayo Clinic in Minnesota, and Johns Hopkins University in Baltimore. On the basis of follow-up periods averaging between 4.4 and 6.3 years, the percentage of men at ten or fifteen years following surgery who would have evidence of cancer recurrence as measured by PSA and by the spread of the cancer (metastases) was calculated. Deaths due to the prostate cancer were also estimated.

The results of the studies are summarized in Table 2 and are consistent with the results of most smaller studies. The Johns Hopkins study included more men who were younger (average age 58) and who had earlier, and thus more curable, stages of cancer. The number of men with nonpalpable cancer in the Johns Hopkins study was 44 percent, compared to only 7 percent in the Mayo Clinic study. In contrast to the other studies, the Johns Hopkins study excluded seventy-five men from follow-up because of evidence of advanced cancer and the need for additional treatment; such exclusions improve recurrence rates.

Given the data, what can be said about outcomes following prostate surgery? It seems evident that recurrence of prostate cancer is not a rare occurrence. At ten years after surgery, at least one quarter of men will have a recurrence of cancer as measured by PSA, and at least 10 percent will have metastases. At ten years, the death rate from prostate cancer is less than 10 percent. Fifteen years after surgery, there is more evidence of cancer, and the death rate from the cancer varies from 10 percent in younger men with less severe disease to 18 percent in older men with more severe disease.

Finally, the surgical treatment of prostate cancer has one striking advantage over all other treatments, which is that it provides men with the most information. After surgery, men know their exact Gleason score based on the entire cancer, not just the biopsy, and they know whether cancer has spread outside the prostate to seminal vesicles or surrounding lymph nodes. And because the entire prostate is removed at surgery, monitoring the postsurgical level of PSA provides an accurate and unambiguous measure of cancer recurrence. Thus, surgical treatment removes many uncertainties from the follow-up; the news may not necessarily be favorable, but at least the patient knows what the news is. Perhaps for these reasons a comparative study of the mental health of men treated by surgery, beam radiation, or watchful waiting reported that the men treated by surgery worried significantly less after treatment than men in the other two groups.[23]

4

Radiation Treatment

After surgery, radiation is the most frequent treatment of prostate cancer in the United States. Its popularity increased after Andy Grove, chairman of Intel, published a 1996 *Fortune* magazine cover story account of why he had selected radiation treatment for his prostate cancer. An analysis of Medicare data found that radioactive seed therapy (brachytherapy) "is replacing radical prostatectomy as the treatment of choice for early-stage prostate cancer."[1] Radiation is, of course, used to treat many forms of cancer. It works by disrupting the deoxyribonucleic acid (DNA) of cancer cells, which grow more rapidly than do normal cells; both types of cells are damaged, but cancer cells are damaged more severely.

Radiation has been used to treat prostate cancer since the early years of the last century. One of the originators of the idea was Alexander Graham Bell. In 1903, while president of the National Geographic Society, Bell wrote to a physician who was treating cancer: "There is no reason why a tiny fragment of radium sealed in a fine glass tube should not be inserted into the very heart of the cancer, thus acting directly upon the diseased material." Bell's suggestion was implemented, and by 1917 reports began to be published on the efficacy of radium, inserted directly into the tumor, for treating prostate cancer.[2] The use of external radiation to treat prostate cancer, called beam therapy, did not become widespread until the 1960s.

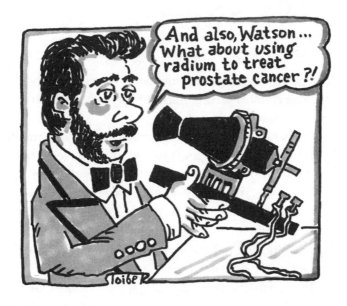

Both forms of radiation treatment—placing the radioactive substance into the cancer, and beaming it into the cancer from outside the body—are widely used. The former is now widely referred to as seed therapy. Officially, it is called interstitial radiotherapy or brachytherapy, "brachy" being the Greek word for *short* and implying that the radiation is placed a short distance from the cancer. The seeds may be implanted permanently or just for several hours; the latter is known as high dose rate (HDR) brachytherapy. Radioactive forms of iodine, palladium, and iridium are presently used to generate the radiation.

Radiation can be beamed into the body from an external source in a variety of ways. The newer methods utilize computers and high-tech equipment to focus the radioactivity sharply on the cancerous tissue, thereby causing less damage to the surrounding tissues and fewer complications. Beam therapy is officially referred to as external beam radiation therapy (EBRT), and the newer variations are called three-dimensional conformal radiation therapy (3DCRT) and intensity-modulated radiotherapy (IMRT). Proton and neutron beam radiation are in experimental stages. The technology of both seed and beam radiation treatment is continuously evolving; it is likely to improve further, especially in the ability to focus the radiation specifically on the cancerous tissue.

Ways Radiation Is Used to Treat Prostate Cancer

A. By placing the radioactive substance directly into the cancer. This is called seed therapy, brachytherapy, or interstitial radiotherapy.
   1. Permanent: Seeds are inserted and left in permanently.
   2. Temporary: Seeds are implanted for several hours, then removed. This is called HDR (high dose rate) brachytherapy and is sometimes referred to as the Andy Grove method, since it was popularized by the Intel chairman.
B. By beaming the radiation into the cancer from outside. This is called external beam radiation therapy, or EBRT.
   1. Three-dimensional conformal radiation therapy (3DCRT): special computers produce a precise focus of the beam.
   2. Intensity-modulated radiotherapy (IMRT): a high-tech version of 3DCRT in which radiation comes from multiple directions.
   3. Conformal proton beam radiation therapy: as above, but using protons rather than X-rays.

WHO ARE GOOD CANDIDATES?

Radiation treatment, like surgical treatment, works best on men with less severe forms of prostate cancer. Ideal candidates are thus men whose tumor is not palpable (stage T1c), or palpable but occupying less than half of one lobe (stage T2a); whose PSA is less than 10; and whose Gleason score is 6 or less. For Gleason scores of 7 or more, seed therapy is not recommended unless it is used together with beam therapy. One study showed that the best candidates for beam therapy are those with the lowest percentages of cancer-positive cores (one third or less) on biopsy; this finding is similar to the recommendation for good candidates for surgical treatment.[3]

A Man Who Chose Beam Therapy

If I have surgery, I'll be inactive for a long time. I'm in good shape for seventy-eight and want to stay that way a while longer. I don't know what side effects I'll have with radiation but I'm optimistic, I feel I'll be able to continue my power walks, travels and work. . . . I need to be in Boulder for an Antarctic workshop May 7 to 9.

—Charles Neider, *Adam's Burden*

Men who do not wish to have surgery or who cannot have surgery for medical reasons are also candidates for radiation therapy. Some men simply do not wish to subject themselves to a major surgical procedure with its attendant risks and extended recovery period. Others have heart, lung, kidney, or other medical conditions that increase the risk of major surgery. Seed therapy requires minor surgery and thus can be carried out on many of these men; beam therapy requires no surgery at all and is often the first choice of such men.

It can also be argued that radiation therapy is a wise choice for older men, especially those with a life expectancy of less than fifteen years. As will be discussed below, the long-term survival of men treated with radiation appears to be as high as that of those treated surgically for at least the first ten years following diagnosis of their cancer; if surgical treatment has an advantage in regard to life expectancy, it probably becomes manifest only after that period. Therefore, if a man is not likely to live more than ten years, it is logical to select a treatment without the burden and complications of prostate surgery. In practice, older men are more likely to choose radiation over surgical treatment; in one study of men in their 70s, radiation was chosen seven times more frequently than surgery.[4]

Finally, beam radiation therapy is increasingly being used for men who have undergone surgical removal of their prostate cancer but in whom, following surgery, it is discovered that not all the

A Man Who Chose a Combination of Seed Therapy
and Beam Therapy

Whatever therapy I chose, I would be willing to accept an increased risk of dying, if I could preserve my sexuality. I also vowed to do whatever I could to avoid becoming a urological cripple. That determination would become my compass, as I worked to set a course in—what was for me—the uncharted wilderness of cancer.

—Michael Dorso, *Seeds of Hope*

cancer was removed (there is a "positive margin," or the cancer has spread through the prostate capsule). A 2005 European study demonstrated definitively that beam therapy following such surgery significantly improved the outcome.[5]

Finally, men may select radiation treatment because they believe that it has fewer side effects, especially incontinence and impotence, than surgical treatment.

Some men are not viable candidates for radiation treatment, especially those with large prostates (over 50 to 60 grams). A normal prostate in a young man weighs approximately 20 grams, then increases gradually as he ages. Large prostates require more seeds, a fact that increases the treatment's side effects. Large prostates are also difficult to irradiate adequately by beam therapy without injuring the surrounding tissues and without leaving untreated areas of the prostate (commonly referred to as "cold spots"). In some cases, the size of large prostates can be reduced by first giving hormone treatment. Many urologists believe that men with diseases of the urinary tract or diseases of the colon, such as ulcerative colitis, are not appropriate candidates for radiation treatment because radiation may exacerbate those diseases. Finally, seed therapy is generally not used for men who have previously had part of their prostate removed surgically to relieve symptoms of BPH; scar tissue complicates the placing of the seeds. For recurrent cancers, seed therapy by itself is not used, although beam therapy is used, often in conjunction with hormone therapy (see Chapter 11).

In the past, seed therapy and beam therapy have each been used by themselves. Today, increasingly, they are being used together or in conjunction with other treatments. This is true not only for advanced cancers but also for early- and intermediate-stage cancers, some of which are currently being treated with both seed and beam therapy or with beam and hormone therapy. Such use of combined treatments remains controversial; some radiation advocates argue that seed or beam radiation therapy by itself is sufficient, while others argue that combined therapy produces better outcomes. The data to resolve this controversy do not yet exist.

THE PROCEDURE

Seed Therapy

Compared to other treatments for prostate cancer, seed therapy is convenient—a major reason for its increasing popularity. Usually, only two outpatient visits are required.

On the first visit, the radiation oncologist places an ultrasound probe, similar to that used in prostate biopsies, in the rectum and then carefully maps the prostate. This allows for a calculation of exactly where seeds should be placed and how many—usually fifty to one hundred—will be needed.

On the second visit, the man is given a regional block (spinal or epidural) or general anesthesia for a procedure that lasts approximately an hour. While he is on his back with his legs elevated and spread, long needles are inserted into the prostate through the perineum, the area between the back of the scrotum and the anus. The radioactive seeds, which are smaller than grains of rice, are inserted into the prostate through the needles. It is vital that the seeds be placed evenly, so that no areas of cancer are left untreated; therefore, ultrasound, CT scans, and/or fluoroscopy are used to guide the placement. An antibiotic is given to minimize the chances of infection.

Following the procedure, the patient is taken to the recovery room for a few hours, then allowed to go home. A urinary catheter is

Lawyers and Seed Therapy

John Blasko, M.D., is a pioneer radiation oncologist in Seattle and a leader in promoting seed therapy. He advises men to take a week off from work following the implantation procedure. He is also quoted as saying: "The only people I send back to work right away are lawyers. These people are used to being a pain in the ass."

—Michael Dorso, *Seeds of Hope*

used during the procedure but is usually removed before discharge. Postoperative pain can be controlled by ice packs and pain pills. A graphic first-person account of this procedure is found in Michael Dorso's *Seeds of Hope*.

Following implantation of the seeds, the patient can resume normal activities within days. One man claimed to have run a half-marathon two weeks after the procedure![1] Most men have some continuing discomfort, including frequency and urgency of urination, abdominal tenderness, and pain in the rectum. These symptoms generally resolve over several weeks, although they may recur later.

After implantation of the seeds, men are mildly radioactive for up to two months. During that time, they are advised not to stand within six feet of a pregnant woman, not to allow small children to sit on their laps, and not to try to conceive a child. Some physicians also ask them to wear a condom during intercourse in case a radioactive seed is expelled with the ejaculate. Modern screening techniques at airports may also detect radiation from the seeds, so men may wish to carry a note from their physician. By the end of the two months, the seeds are no longer radioactive and remain in the man's prostate for the rest of his life.

The follow-up for men with seed therapy generally consists of an appointment two to three weeks after implantation to assess the dose of radiation. Another appointment a month later assesses

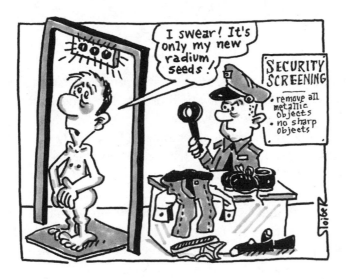

Recovery from Seed Therapy

As I was dressing, I realized that my scrotum was twice its normal size, and deep purple! That startled me. I had an ache in my groin, but my scrotum looked like I should be feeling serious pain!

That evening wasn't too bad. My job was to lie in the hotel bed with an ice bag in my crotch. Pain pills made it tolerable as I watched TV. I had a constant urge to urinate, and was up frequently trying to pee, but with limited success. Sometime in the middle of the night I passed an obstructing blood clot through my penis—followed by a surge of pent up urine. Now that got my attention! That was probably the most uncomfortable event of the entire therapy.

—Michael Dorso, *Seeds of Hope*

Beam Therapy

Here in this surrealistic chamber was the best that modern medicine had to offer. It would be here that I must fight my battle with the killer in my groin. . . .

There I was, alone in this temple of technology. Everyone else had fled the radiation that would soon be flooding the room. A mental image of a sacrificial lamb on the altar flashed through my mind. . . .

Even though I knew I would feel nothing when the radiation hit me, I had to resist the urge to cringe. I felt a need to lighten up, as I lay there staring up at the x-ray machine. I chose to address the one-eyed Cyclops.

"Take me to your leader, alien!"

It must have heard me! Suddenly it was alive and buzzing.

—Michael Dorso, *Seeds of Hope*

possible complications. A PSA and rectal exam are usually done every four to six months for the next five years, then annually.

Beam Radiation

The procedure for beam therapy is substantially more onerous than for seed therapy, despite the fact that beam therapy involves no anesthesia, surgery, or pain and is performed completely on an outpatient basis.

Before beam therapy can be started, several visits to the hospital's radiology department are required. During these visits, a cradle-like cast is made of the man's body; during each radiation treatment, he will lie in that cast to ensure that he is absolutely immobile and unable to move during the treatments. Small black tattoos are placed on the lower abdomen so that the radiation beam can be correctly aligned each time. The lower abdomen is carefully mapped by putting a contrast material into the bladder and rectum and taking X-ray pictures of it; this helps ensure that the radiation beam will be directed precisely at the prostate and not at another organ.

The actual treatments are given five days a week for five to nine weeks. Thus, men must be prepared to follow a rigid treatment schedule for several weeks and are not allowed to miss a treatment. This regimen may pose no problem for men who work in metropolitan areas where they can stop by the hospital each day on the way to work. But for men who live in more rural areas, it may involve staying in a hotel in the city for the entire treatment period.

The treatments themselves are quick and painless. The man lies in his custom-made cast on the X-ray table in a semidarkened room for about fifteen minutes. Depending on the specific type of beam therapy being used, the huge X-ray machine may be stationary overhead or it may move during the treatment. Laser beams, often from several directions, give the room a Star Wars ambience; one half expects to see Han Solo and Luke Skywalker come through the door.

COMPLICATIONS

Two minor side effects of beam therapy are pubic hair loss and fatigue. The hair loss may be temporary or permanent, but the radiation does not affect hair on the head. Fatigue, which may be marked, usually begins three to four weeks after the treatment course begins. Exercise can help; one study reported that men who walked for thirty minutes each day during the treatment period experienced less radiation fatigue.[6]

Symptoms of urinary dysfunction are common in men who undergo radiation treatments, both immediately following the treatment and months or even years later. Frequency, urgency, pain on urination, trouble starting the urinary stream, narrowing of the stream, and inability to empty the bladder completely are all common. Relatively less frequent are symptoms of incontinence.

Men undergoing beam therapy are assessed for urinary symptoms a number of times. At five to ten months after treatment, 12 percent of men complained of frequency, and 18 percent of urgency. Two to four years later, these symptoms of urinary irritation continued to be reported by 15 to 44 percent of men in different studies, with severe symptoms in 2 or 3 percent. One study that assessed thirty-nine men an average of thirteen years after beam therapy reported that half of them continued to report urinary symptoms, especially episodes of blood in their urine (hematuria).[7] It can be argued, however, that these men were treated with technologically earlier versions of beam therapy that were less focused on the prostate and did more damage to the bladder.

For seed therapy, reports of irritative urinary symptoms are similar to, if not more severe than, for beam therapy. One study that directly compared the two forms of radiation approximately two years after treatment reported that those who had undergone seed therapy had significantly more urinary symptoms. Several studies have reported that men who are treated with a combination of seed and beam therapies have more urinary symptoms than men treated with either therapy alone; this finding is not surprising since the combination yields a higher dose of radiation than either therapy alone.[8]

It is important to note that although irritative urinary symptoms are common, symptoms of urinary incontinence are relatively unusual in men treated with radiation. One large study reported that only 4 percent of men were still wearing pads five years after beam therapy.[9] The irritative urinary symptoms can often be ameliorated with medication.

Symptoms of impotence and erectile dysfunction are common in men who undergo either beam or seed therapy. Rates of impotence immediately following beam therapy are low but then increase progressively during the following five years to 50 to 60 percent, owing to radiation effects on the nerves and small arteries going to the penis.

The same pattern is seen after seed therapy, with a slow increase in erectile dysfunction in the first five years after treatment. Pain during orgasm (26 to 40 percent) and blood in the ejaculate (15 to 17 percent) have also been described following seed therapy. Although seed therapy reputedly causes less impotence than beam therapy, two of the three studies that directly compared the two treatments reported more impotence for men who had undergone seed therapy, while the third study reported impotence to be slightly higher following beam therapy.

It has been suggested that drugs like sildenafil (Viagra) are more

Urinary Complications

I've also had to deal with an irritable bladder. Mine wasn't happy being caught in the radiation bathing my pelvis. It now seems to register *full* at three ounces, and with unseemly insistence. That makes it difficult to sit through a movie or more than a hundred miles in a car. A shopping trip has to be planned with a pit stop in mind. I'm certainly becoming aware of where all the bathrooms are in town.

—Michael Dorso, *Seeds of Hope*

likely to be effective in improving erections in men who have had seed therapy than in those who underwent beam therapy. There is also evidence, as would be expected, that men who undergo a combination of beam and seed therapy have more impotence than men undergoing either treatment alone. Two studies that compared older and newer forms of beam and seed therapies both reported lower rates of impotence with the newer forms of radiation; other complications may decrease as well.[10]

Bowel dysfunction is a third major complication of radiation treatment for prostate cancer. This dysfunction includes frequency (diarrhea), urgency that may lead to fecal soiling, cramping, pain in the rectum or painful hemorrhoids, and bleeding. Such symptoms can often be treated with medication and decrease over time in most patients.

In one study at five to ten months following beam therapy, one third of men had bowel frequency and urgency, 18 percent had bleeding, and 16 percent had cramping. A study five years after treatment reported that 16 percent of men were continuing to have diarrhea, and 13 percent to have rectal bleeding. A study of men thirteen years after beam therapy found that 13 percent were still experiencing some rectal bleeding.[11]

Although rare, another bowel complication of radiation to the prostate is rectal cancer. A 2005 study found that beam radiation,

Bowel Complications

Mornings are the worst time, because of bowel movements. Even on a low-bulk diet, I have two or three each morning, and the anus burns fiercely both during the movement and for a couple of hours afterwards. The pain is fatiguing. . . .

The oncoming of a bowel movement is itself unpleasant, and very different from a normal oncoming one. I feel a pervasive, increasing malaise, then increasing anxiety. Only later do I feel signals in the bowel, which come suddenly and urgently while my sphincter warns me I lack normal control over it.

—Charles Neider, *Adam's Burden*

compared to surgery, increased the chances of developing rectal cancer by 70 percent.[12] This figure was widely reported in the medical news media. It is crucial to put such reports in proper perspective. In the study, the chances of developing rectal cancer among men treated with beam therapy was 1 in 246 cases, compared with 1 in 386 cases among men not treated with beam therapy; thus, the risk of rectal cancer increased modestly but not enough to be an overriding factor in selecting treatment.

Studies of rectal complications following seed therapy, although less numerous, report similar findings. In one study five years following treatment, 9 percent of the men were experiencing rectal bleeding. Two studies have compared bowel dysfunction in men who had beam or seed therapy; one of them reported more dysfunction with beam therapy, the other reported the opposite.[13]

There is broad consensus that higher doses of radiation, whether by seeds or by beam, lead to more complications. In one study, higher doses of radiation produced urinary symptoms in 13 percent and rectal symptoms in 14 percent of men five years after treatment, whereas the comparable figures for lower doses of radiation were 4 percent and 5 percent.[14] All comparisons between seed and beam therapies are tentative, since both forms of radiation treatment are still being developed.

Outcome

Assessing the outcome of radiation treatment for prostate cancer is both difficult and confusing. The ultimate outcome measure for the treatment of all forms of cancer is the number of people who die from it, but prostate deaths may not occur until ten, fifteen, or more years after treatment. Because the average age of men with prostate cancer who are treated with radiation has traditionally been older than that of men treated with surgery, many will die from other causes before living long enough to ascertain whether or not their prostate cancer would have killed them.

In lieu of using death as an outcome measure, most researchers on radiation treatment use a rising PSA level, as do those who measure the outcome of surgical treatment. However, there is a major difference: Following surgical removal of the prostate, the PSA level is expected to drop to zero; following radiation treatment, this is not always the case. Radiation is expected to kill all the cancer cells, but not necessarily all the normal prostate cells. The same is true in radiation treatments for cancers of the breast or pituitary gland; radiation is expected to kill all cancer cells but not all normal cells, so the breast and pituitary continue to function after radiation treatments have been completed.

Following radiation treatment for prostate cancer, the PSA is expected to fall, but the level to which it is expected to fall is widely debated. Some researchers say it should become less than 1.0, others 0.5, and others 0.3. In an attempt to establish a standard, the American Society for Therapeutic Radiology and Oncology (ASTRO) decreed in 1997 that, following the fall of the PSA to its lowest level (nadir), a recurrence of prostate cancer should be said to have occurred when the PSA then rises on three consecutive measurements. In practice, the descent of the PSA to its nadir after radiation treatment may take two or more years. Since the PSA is usually measured only two or three times per year, it is often not until three, four, or more years after radiation treatment that the failure of the treatment becomes evident.

Assessing the recurrence of cancer following radiation treatment is still more complicated, however, because of what is called the PSA bounce. In approximately one third of men treated with radiation, PSA levels increase one to three years after treatment, then return to a lower level. This rise does *not* signify the recurrence of cancer but is instead thought to be caused by a delayed release of PSA from irradiated cancer cells. The PSA increase associated with the bounce may last for as long as a year. During this time, there is no way to tell whether the PSA increase is merely a PSA bounce that has no clinical significance, or whether it indicates a failure of radiation treatment and a recurrence of the cancer. If it is a PSA bounce, it will go back down; if not, it will continue to rise.

Despite the problems in assessing the effectiveness of radiation treatment using the PSA, there is strong evidence that the lower the PSA goes after radiation, the less are the chances of recurrence. In one study, men whose PSA was 1.0 or lower following beam therapy had only a 4 percent chance of metastases eight years later, whereas men whose PSA did not go below 2.0 had a 39 percent chance of having metastases eight years later. In another study, men whose PSA was 0.2 or less had only a 1 percent chance of having cancer recurrence eight years later, compared to a 16 percent chance for those with higher PSAs.[15] Thus, the absolute level of the PSA nadir following radiation treatment is important in predicting recurrence.

As noted in Chapter 2, another significant predictor of outcome following beam radiation therapy is the pretreatment PSA velocity. Men who had had PSA increases of 2.0 or more in the years prior to the diagnosis of their prostate cancers had a much higher rate of recurrence and death, compared to men who had had PSA increases of less than 2.0.[16]

Comparing the outcomes of different studies of radiation treatment also generates problems. Some studies use the ASTRO guidelines cited above, while other studies modify those guidelines or use an absolute PSA nadir, such as 1.0 or 0.5. Statistical problems are abundant: some studies use the actual numbers for the follow-up period and others estimate future numbers based on the follow-up period (actuarial numbers).

A study may follow men for five years after treatment and then estimate the ten-year recurrence rate based on the findings from the

Table 3. Outcome of Seed Therapy: Percentage of Patients with Evidence of Cancer Recurrence as Measured by Rising PSA

Study	Number of men	Average follow-up period	Recurrence rate	Period at which recurrence is estimated	Clinical information
Grado et al., 1998 Scottsdale, Ariz.	392	2.5 years	20%	5 years	median age 70.4 20% Gleason ≥7 median PSA 7.3
Ragde et al., 2000 Seattle	147	12.2 years	34%	10 years	average age 70.5 0% Gleason ≥7 average PSA 8.8
Beyer and Brachman, 2000 Scottsdale, Ariz.	695	4.3 years	29%	5 years	median age 74 16% Gleason ≥7 31% PSA >10
Blasko et al., 2000 Seattle	230	3.5 years	18%	9 years	median age 69 40% Gleason ≥7 median PSA 7.3
Grimm et al., 2001 Seattle	125	4.3 years	13%	10 years	median age 70 0% Gleason ≥7 22% PSA >10

SOURCE: G. L. Grado, T. R. Larson, C. S. Balch, et al., Actuarial disease-free survival after prostate cancer brachytherapy using interactive techniques with biplane ultrasound and fluoroscopic guidance, *International Journal of Radiation Oncology, Biology, Physics* 42 (1998): 289–298; H. Ragde, L. J. Korb, A.-A. Elgamal, et al., Modern prostate brachytherapy: Prostate specific antigen results in 219 patients with up to 12 years of observed follow-up, *Cancer* 89 (2000): 135–141; D. C. Beyer and D. G. Brachman, Failure free survival following brachytherapy alone for prostate cancer: Comparison with external beam radiotherapy, *Radiotherapy and Oncology* 57 (2000): 263–267; J. C. Blasko, P. D. Grimm, J. E. Sylvester, et al., Palladium-103 brachytherapy for prostate carcinoma, *International Journal of Radiation Oncology, Biology, Physics* 46 (2000): 839–850; P. D. Grimm, J. C. Blasko, J. E. Sylvester, et al., 10-year biochemical (prostate-specific antigen) control of prostate cancer with 125I brachytherapy, *International Journal of Radiation Oncology, Biology, Physics* 51 (2001): 31–40.

Table 4. Outcome of Beam Therapy: Percentage of Patients with
Evidence of Cancer Recurrence as Measured by Rising PSA

Study	Number of men	Average follow-up period	Recurrence rate	Period at which recurrence is estimated	Clinical information
Kupelian et al., 1997 Cleveland	253	3.5 years	43%	5 years	median age 71 31% Gleason ≥7 58% PSA >10
Beyer and Brachman, 2000 Scottsdale, Ariz.	1,527	3.4 years	31%	5 years	median age 74 26% Gleason ≥7 54% PSA >10
Zelefsky et al., 2001 New York	1,100	5.0 years	15% low risk 45% int. risk 62% high risk	5 years	average age 69 risk defined by Gleason score, PSA, and stage
Hanlon et al., 2002 Philadelphia	615	5.3 years	30% by PSA 7% metastases	5.3 years	average age 69 22% Gleason ≥7 average PSA 15

Klein and Kupelian, 2003 Cleveland	578	4.3 years	30%	8 years	38% Gleason ≥7 42% PSA >10
Zeitman et al., 2004 Boston	205	8.6 years	51% by PSA 18% metastases	10 years	average age 72 31% Gleason ≥7 48% PSA >10
D'Amico et al., 2004 Boston	104	4.5 years	22%	5 years	median age 73 74% Gleason ≥7 median PSA 11

SOURCE: P. Kupelian, J. Katcher, H. Levin, et al., External beam radiotherapy versus radical prostatectomy for clinical stage T1–2 prostate cancer: Therapeutic implications of stratification by pretreatment PSA levels and biopsy Gleason scores, *Cancer Journal from Scientific American* 3 (1997): 78–87; D. C. Beyer and D. G. Brachman, Failure free survival following brachytherapy alone for prostate cancer: Comparison with external beam radiotherapy, *Radiotherapy and Oncology* 57 (2000): 263–267; M. J. Zelefsky, Z. Fuks, M. Hunt, et al., High dose radiation delivered by intensity modulated conformal radiotherapy improves the outcome of localized prostate cancer, *Journal of Urology* 166 (2001): 876–881; A. L. Hanlon, H. Diratzouian, G. E. Hanks, et al., Posttreatment prostate-specific antigen nadir highly predictive of distant failure and death from prostate cancer, *International Journal of Radiation Oncology, Biology, Physics* 53 (2002): 297–303; A. L. Zeitman, C. S. Chung, J. J. Coen, et al., 10-year outcome for men with localized prostate cancer treated with external radiation therapy: Results of a cohort study, *Journal of Urology* 171 (2004): 210–214; A. V. D'Amico, J. Manola, M. Loffredo, et al., 6-month androgen suppression plus radiation therapy vs radiation therapy alone for patients with clinically localized prostate cancer, *Journal of the American Medical Association* 292 (2004): 821–827.

first five years. It is known that the shorter the period of real follow-up, the less accurate the actuarial estimates are apt to be. It has also been demonstrated that actual and actuarial numbers may differ considerably. In addition to these problems, different studies of radiation treatment outcomes include men of different average ages, different severity of cancers, different types of seed and beam therapies, and different amounts of radiation.

If we keep these serious limitations in mind, what are the results of radiation outcome studies for prostate cancer? The major studies are summarized in Tables 3–5. Following seed therapy (Table 3) the recurrence of cancer, as measured by a rising PSA, is approximately 15 to 30 percent at five years posttreatment and appears to be approximately the same at ten years, depending in part on the number of men in the study with high PSAs or high Gleason scores. However, most men in these studies had less severe forms of prostate cancer; in the five studies cited, an average of only 15 percent of the men had pretreatment Gleason scores of 7 or higher. Thus, most men in these studies would be expected to have a low rate of recurrence.

For beam therapy (Table 4), the recurrence of cancer, as measured by a rising PSA, is approximately 25 to 40 percent at five years posttreatment, and approximately 35 to 50 percent at ten years. The men in these studies had significantly more advanced cancers at the time of treatment than the men in the seed therapy studies; for example, approximately half of them had Gleason scores of 7 or higher.

Men treated with a combination of seed and beam therapy (Table 5) appeared to have a comparatively favorable outcome, similar to that for seed therapy. As noted previously, some researchers believe that adding beam therapy to seed therapy for men with low- and intermediate-grade cancers improves the outcome; other researchers disagree.

In summary, three facts stand out. First, multiple studies have demonstrated that the higher the dose of radiation given, the lower the recurrence rate.

Second, it is evident that the higher the dose of radiation given, the more serious the complications affecting the urinary tract, the ability to have erections, and the rectal function. These two facts put men and their oncologists squarely between a rock and a hard place.

The third fact is that the selection of patients for any outcome

Table 5. Outcome of Seed and Beam Therapies When Given Together: Percentage of Patients with Evidence of Cancer Recurrence as Measured by Rising PSA

Study	Number of men	Average follow-up period	Recurrence rate	Period at which recurrence is estimated	Clinical information
Grado et al., 1998 Scottsdale, Ariz.	62	2.0 years	28%	5 years	median age 70.2 37% Gleason ≥7 median PSA 8.7
Ragde et al., 2000 Seattle	75	12.2 years	21%	10 years	median age 70.4 18% Gleason ≥7 average PSA 14.7
Critz et al., 2000 Decatur, Ga.	689	4.0 years	12%	5 years	median age 66 23% Gleason ≥7 27% PSA >10
Merrick et al., 2004 Wheeling, W.Va.	119	5.4 years	2%	7 years	median age 58.1 82% low risk by Gleason, PSA, and stage

SOURCE: G. L. Grado, T. R. Larson, C. S. Balch, et al., Actuarial disease-free survival after prostate cancer brachytherapy using interactive techniques with biplane ultrasound and fluoroscopic guidance, International Journal of Radiation Oncology, Biology, Physics 42 (1998): 289–298; H. Ragde, L. J. Korb, A.-A. Elgamal, et al., Modern prostate brachytherapy: Prostate specific antigen results in 219 patients with up to 12 years of observed follow-up, Cancer 89 (2000): 135–141; F. A. Critz, W. H. Williams, A. K. Levinson, et al., Simultaneous irradiation for prostate cancer: Intermediate results with modern techniques, Journal of Urology 164 (2000): 738–743; G. S. Merrick, W. M. Butler, K. E. Wallner, et al., Permanent interstitial brachytherapy in younger patients with clinically organ-confined prostate cancer, Urology 64 (2004):754–759.

study profoundly affects the results. At one end of the patient-selection spectrum is a study in which 67 percent of the men had a Gleason score of at least 7 or a PSA of at least 10, with 28 percent having PSA scores of over 20; a five-year recurrence rate of 43 percent is not surprising among men with such serious forms of cancer. At the other end of the spectrum is a study that included only younger men (average age 58.1) with less serious forms of cancer. This study reported a recurrence rate of 2 percent at seven years posttreatment. *In evaluating claims of better results for individual treatment centers or specific treatments, we must always examine the selection of men who were included in the treatment study.*

One final measure of outcome is how satisfied men are retrospectively with the treatment they chose. Relatively few studies have been made on this question, and most men say they are satisfied with their decision. One study reported that, approximately three years after treatment, fifteen of ninety-six men wished they had chosen a different treatment. Those who were dissatisfied included three of fifty-six (5 percent) who had had surgery; one of eleven (10 percent) who was pursuing watchful waiting; three of sixteen (19 percent) who had chosen beam therapy; and eight of thirteen (62 percent) who had undergone seed therapy.[17] These numbers are small and the differences not statistically significant; more such studies are needed in order to obtain a useful measure of outcome.

CHAPTER

5

Hormone Treatment

Testosterone, the male sex hormone produced by the testicles, stimulates the growth of prostate cancers. It was discovered more than a century ago that surgical removal of the testicles—castration—improves symptoms for men with advanced prostate cancer. Charles Huggins, a urologist at the University of Chicago, undertook experiments in 1941 to bring about the same effect by giving men with prostate cancer female sex hormones to block testosterone. This work, which in essence produces a chemical castration, was the first successful treatment of any form of cancer using medication. For his research, Huggins was awarded a Nobel Prize in Medicine in 1966.

For the past half-century, hormone treatment has been commonly used to treat prostate cancer, mostly for advanced cases in which the cancer has spread to the bones or other organs. In the 1990s, the use of hormones to treat prostate cancer broadened to include earlier stages of cancer, especially in conjunction with radiation beam therapy. In 1989, only 10 percent of men being treated by beam therapy were also given hormone treatment; by 2001, this figure had increased to 75 percent.[1]

The reduction of testosterone by hormone treatment both slows the growth of cancer cells and kills them. The oldest and most

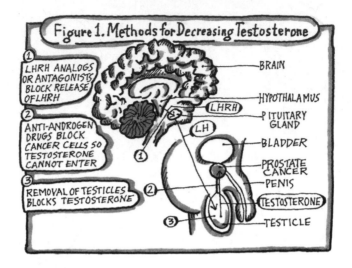

Figure 1. Methods for Decreasing Testosterone

① LHRH ANALOGS OR ANTAGONISTS BLOCK RELEASE OF LHRH

② ANTI-ANDROGEN DRUGS BLOCK CANCER CELLS SO TESTOSTERONE CANNOT ENTER

③ REMOVAL OF TESTICLES BLOCKS TESTOSTERONE

BRAIN
HYPOTHALAMUS
PITUITARY GLAND
BLADDER
PROSTATE CANCER
PENIS
TESTOSTERONE
TESTICLE

direct method of reducing testosterone is surgical castration. Another method is giving a drug that blocks testosterone from getting into the cancer cells. Such drugs are called antiandrogens; examples are bicalutamide (Casodex) and flutamide (Eulexin).

A third method of reducing testosterone is cutting off the hormone (called luteinizing hormone, or LH) that stimulates the testicles to produce testosterone. This LH is made by the pituitary gland in response to instructions from the hypothalamus in the brain. A group of drugs called luteinizing hormone–releasing hormone (or LHRH) agonists and antagonists trick the hypothalamus into not sending instructions to the pituitary. The pituitary in turn fails to send LH to the testicles, so no testosterone is produced. Leuprolide (Lupron) and goserelin (Zoladex) are examples of LHRH agonists, and abarelix (Plenaxis) is an example of an LHRH antagonist. Figure 1 illustrates these chemical methods for reducing testosterone.

WHO ARE GOOD CANDIDATES?

The best candidates for hormone therapy are men whose prostate is large or whose cancer has spread locally, beyond the prostate. This treatment is also used for men whose cancer has spread distantly to bones (see Chapter 11). Hormones are routinely used for men whose cancer has spread locally to lymph nodes near the prostate, and they are being used increasingly often, together with radiation, for men

---

Michael Milken's Prostate Cancer

In 1993, Michael Milken, a forty-six-year-old former Wall Street financier, was diagnosed with prostate cancer. His PSA was 24, and cancer had already spread to his lymph nodes but not to his bones. He was immediately started on combined hormone therapy, consisting of both an antiandrogen and an LHRH agonist. Within six months, his PSA had fallen to 3, and he was given radiation treatment. Using continuing hormone treatment and strict dietary control, Milken's cancer has continued to remain in remission.

—adapted from Leon Jaroff, The man's cancer,
Time, April 1, 1996

---

who have high-grade cancers (such as Gleason types 8, 9, and 10) that are likely to spread.

In men who have very large prostates, hormone treatment shrinks the prostate so that seed or beam radiation therapy will be more effective. Finally, hormones may be used as the only treatment for elderly men with prostate cancer who are unable or unwilling to undergo surgical or radiation treatments.

Men with low- and intermediate-grade prostate cancers are not thought to be viable candidates for hormone treatment. However, hormones are being used more and more frequently in such cases, despite the fact that no studies demonstrate that they are of any value. Some physicians start men on hormone treatment immediately after their diagnosis while the patients are deciding what definitive treatment they wish to have; the side effects of such treatment must be weighed against the dubious benefits of its use.

THE PROCEDURE

The earliest form of hormone treatment, removal of the testicles, can be done surgically on an outpatient basis. It is officially called an

Drugs Used for Hormone Treatment of Prostate Cancer

Antiandrogens (taken as pills)
bicalutamide (Casodex)
flutamide (Eulexin)
nilutamide (Nilandron, Anandron)
LHRH Agonists and Antagonists (given by injection)
leuprolide (Lupron, Eligard, Viadur implant)
goserelin (Zoladex)
triptorelin (Trelstar)
abarelix (Plenaxis)

orchiectomy, from the Greek word *orchis,* for "testicle." The proce-dure ensures that no testosterone will be available to stimulate pros-tate cancer cells. Its advantages include not having to take monthly injections, and its low cost compared to other forms of hormone therapy; its main disadvantage is that it is permanent and thus can-not be used like intermittent hormone therapy to decrease side ef-fects. Historically, castration has been carried out for other reasons as well. Castrated men were called eunuchs in ancient Persia, India, and China and were put in charge of harems; often, they rose to govern-mental positions of high authority. Castrati have also been valued for their singing voices. Many men today elect methods of testoster-one suppression other than orchiectomy for prostate cancer. Surgical castration is a deeply emotional issue for men, and there are very few harem positions available to provide consolation!

Antiandrogen drugs are taken orally. Flutamide (Eulexin) must be taken three times a day, but the others can be taken once daily. The LHRH agonists, by contrast, must be taken as injections, usually in the buttock. They can be given once a month or every three months; leuprolide (Lupron) has an additional formulation that can be injected every four months. A different formulation of leupro-lide, Viadur, can be implanted under the skin and lasts for one year. Abarelix (Plenaxis) is an LHRH antagonist; its action is different from

Drug Costs

The following are approximate monthly costs of the hormone treatments commonly used for prostate cancer, as reported in 2004 by the *Medical Letter* (46:22–23). Many men take both an LHRH blocker and an antiandrogen. In 2004, Medicare decreased the reimbursement rate to doctors for administering the LHRH blockers; the expense for patients has increased accordingly.

Antiandrogens

bicalutamide (Casodex)	$417
flutamide (Eulexin)	$444
nilutamide (Nilandron, Anandron)	$344

LHRH blockers

leuprolide	
Lupron Depot	$685
Eligard	$612
Viadur	$474
goserelin (Zoladex)	$470
triptorelin (Trelstar Depot)	$420
abarelix (Plenaxis)	$944

that of the agonists, but the results are the same. Because of serious side effects, it is given only to men who cannot take the other drugs. The cost of the antiandrogens and the LHRH blockers, several hundred dollars per month, is covered by most medical insurance plans. Some companies making these drugs have programs that supply them to men who are not covered by insurance.

In the past, diethylstilbestrol (DES) was used to suppress testosterone. It is no longer used because of its side effects. Ketoconazole (Nizoral) and megestrol (Megace) are occasionally used, and other drugs are being developed.

Many controversial issues exist with regard to how hormone treatments should be given. One debate concerns which is more effective, an antiandrogen or an LHRH blocker. Another addresses whether the two types of hormone treatment should be given together (as is commonly done) as a "combined androgen blockade." Other issues include the optimal duration of treatment when using hormones at the same time as radiation treatment, and whether the hormone treatment is most effective if given before, during, or after the radiation treatment.

In addition, concerning hormone treatment for men whose surgical or radiation treatment has failed, it is debated whether hormone treatment should be started as soon as the PSA increases or whether it is better to wait until clinical or radiologic signs indicate that the cancer is actually spreading. There is also lively argument about whether hormone treatment should be intermittently stopped, to give the body a chance to recover, or whether it is most effective if given continuously. Intermittent hormone therapy consists of starting hormone treatment when the PSA exceeds, say, 4.0; continuing it until it falls below 1.0; then stopping until the PSA again exceeds 4.0. Preliminary studies suggest that intermittent therapy produces outcomes similar to continuous hormone treatment but with fewer side effects; therefore it is being increasingly used.[2]

COMPLICATIONS

Hormone treatment has serious side effects. A man should be started on hormone therapy only when it is likely that the benefits of treatment will outweigh the side effects. The most important side effects are the following:

• *Hot flashes*: Similar to those experienced by women undergoing menopause, these occur in approximately half of men on hormone therapy. They vary from mild flushing to drenching perspiration and may last from a minute to an hour. Medications, including megestrol (Megace), low-dose estrogen compounds, venlafaxine (Effexor), gabapentin (Neurontin), and paroxetine (Paxil), may provide relief.

• *Breast tenderness and enlargement*: This symptom occurs in approximately one third of men and is more common in those taking antiandrogens, especially after being on the medication for several months.

Hot Flashes

"Menopause" is just another word in the dictionary for most men. While some make a token effort to research and empathize with their mates, in most cases, men feel that it's enough for them to show tolerance as women "go through the change." It's difficult for men to relate. Few even try.

Sometimes nature has a way of putting the proverbial shoe on the other foot. I've learned the hard way. Even in the biting cold of winter, I find myself having to sleep with both a ceiling fan and a floor fan on trying to cool the hot flashes that I experience throughout the night.

—Charles Williams, *That Black Men Might Live*

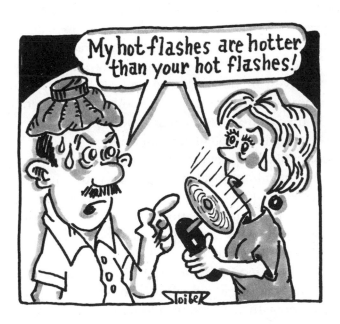

Breast Effects

It is now seven months since I began my hormone suppression therapy. I had no idea that I would miss my testosterone so much. I've nicknamed this therapy *Reverse Steroids*. This is not just some therapeutic idea that is to be taken lightly. My body is definitely changing. My breasts are enlarging. If this gets any worse, I'll need to try on some training bras!

—Michael Dorso, *Seeds of Hope*

• *Impotence*: Difficulty with erections occurs in almost all men on hormone therapy, especially men who have undergone orchiectomy or are taking LHRH blockers. Impotence occurs somewhat less frequently in men taking antiandrogens, particularly in the initial months of treatment, since these men continue to produce testosterone.

• *Decreased libido*: Following surgical and radiation treatments for prostate cancer, erections are frequently impaired because of damage to nerves, arteries, and veins, but the libido remains intact. Following hormone therapy, however, both erections and libido are affected. In the first instance, men may be impotent and care; in the second, they may be impotent and not care.

• *Osteoporosis*: This is one of the most serious side effects of hormone treatment, and its incidence increases with time. Studies have shown that men on hormone therapy lose 8 to 10 percent of their bone mass in the first two years of treatment, then approximately 2 percent per year thereafter. Consequently, 20 percent of men on long-term hormone treatment experience a bone fracture within five years.[3] This risk can be minimized by regular exercise, calcium, and vitamin D supplementation. Medications called biphosphonates can offset the effects of hormone therapy and rebuild bones; the best-studied drugs are pamidronate (Aredia), alendronate (Fosamax), and zoledronic acid (Zometa). In 2006, however, reports linked these drugs to serious problems in the jawbone. Men who will be taking hormone therapy for several years should have a baseline bone mineral density scan.

Lost Libido

Some changes have not been so subtle. It's been at least six months since Sherry and I were able to have sexual inter-course. It's as if the wires from my brain to my penis have been disconnected. Come to think of it, that's exactly what has happened! I embrace my wife, and nothing stirs in my loins. Fortunately, I've had a concomitant loss of libido, so I don't seem to miss the sex too much.

—Michael Dorso, *Seeds of Hope*

• *Fatigue*: Approximately half of men taking hormone treat-ments experience fatigue and weakness. The cause may be a loss of muscle mass or anemia, both of which may be side effects of the treatment. Regular exercise can help, and anemia should be treated if it occurs.

• *Mental changes*: Some men on hormone treatment experience increased moodiness. Depression has been frequently reported, but it is unclear whether it is attributable to the hormones, the side ef-fects of the hormones, or the cancer itself. Earlier studies suggested that men on hormone treatment have problems with their memory, but a 2003 study found that, contrary to what was expected, the memories of the men on hormones significantly improved.[4]

• *Worsening of symptoms*: When LHRH analog drugs are first started, they produce a brief outpouring of testosterone that may temporarily worsen the prostate cancer symptoms. This sequence can be especially problematic if the cancer has already spread to the bones. The temporary worsening of symptoms is called a flair; it can be blocked by giving an antiandrogen for at least one week prior to the first injection of the LHRH analog.

Other side effects of hormone treatments may include weight gain, elevation of cholesterol, diarrhea (with flutamide), and impair-ment of night vision (with nilutamide). In addition, hormone treat-ments affect the PSA level, causing it to become less useful as a mea-sure of recurrence of the cancer.

Benefits of Hormone Treatment

The [hormone] treatment had one unexpected benefit: it improved my driving. No kidding! It made me less aggressive, which is one of the accidental blessings of the whole thing. I don't know if it was the hormonal therapy, or just facing my mortality, but I found myself less judgmental than I used to be.

—Don, in David Bostwick et al., *Prostate Cancer*

OUTCOME

Despite the significant side effects of hormone treatment, it can be effective in treating prostate cancer. For men with metastatic disease where the cancer has spread to other sites, hormone therapy may improve both the quality and quantity of their lives (see Chapter 11). For men with intermediate and advanced grades where the cancer has spread locally or is at high risk of doing so, hormone treatment in conjunction with radiation is proving to be highly effective.

The benefits of hormone therapy show up in a study carried out by the European Organization for Research and Treatment of Cancer (EORTC). A total of 415 men with prostate cancer were randomly assigned to be treated either by beam therapy alone or by beam therapy plus three years of hormone treatment with an LHRH agonist. Only 11 percent of the men had early stages of cancer; the remainder had intermediate or advanced stages, many with local extension of the cancer outside the prostate but without distant spread. At a follow-up period 5.5 years later, men treated with the combination of beam plus hormone had less evidence of clinical disease (26 percent versus 60 percent), less evidence of distant metastases (10 percent versus 29 percent), and fewer deaths due to prostate cancer (12 versus 42) than men treated by beam therapy alone.[5]

A similar study was carried out by the Radiation Therapy Oncology Group (RTOG), a consortium of U.S. cancer treatment centers. A total of 945 men, all of whom had prostate cancer that had spread locally, were randomly assigned to receive either beam therapy alone or beam therapy plus an LHRH agonist that was started during the last week of radiation and continued indefinitely. At the end of six years, men treated with the combined therapy had fewer distant metastases (27 percent versus 37 percent) and fewer deaths from their cancer (65 versus 80). Other RTOG studies have demonstrated that a combination of radiation plus hormone therapy is more effective than radiation alone for men with very large prostate cancers and for those with Gleason scores of 8 to 10. Still another U.S. study reported that radiation plus hormone therapy, compared to radiation alone, benefited men with a Gleason score of 7 or more and a PSA of at least 10.[6]

It seems established, therefore, that adjuvant hormone therapy, when given with radiation beam therapy, improves the outcome in some men with intermediate and advanced stages of prostate cancer. The optimal type and duration of hormone treatment and the dose of radiation are still being debated; several ongoing trials are attempting to answer these questions.

It is less clearly established, however, that adjuvant hormone therapy is useful for men with earlier stages of prostate cancer. Nine ongoing studies that combine hormone treatment with radical prostatectomy, radiation, or watchful waiting are trying to resolve this issue. The largest of these, the Bicalutamide Early Prostate Cancer Study, is following 8,113 men in North America, Europe, Israel, Australia, and Mexico; its preliminary findings suggest that hormone therapy may be useful in this group.[7] If any benefit is demonstrated, it will have to be carefully weighed against the side effects of taking hormones.

When hormone therapy has been given to men with prostate cancer prior to surgery, it has not shown any benefit.[8] Many surgeons, in fact, note that hormone treatment prior to surgery can distort normal anatomical landmarks and makes the surgery more difficult.

6

Cryotherapy

The idea of killing cancer cells by freezing them has a long history. The technique is widely used for some forms of skin cancer. Cryotherapy, also called cryoablation, was first tried for prostate cancer in the 1960s, but the results were disappointing. This approach was revived in the early 1990s and, with improved technology, has gradually gained adherents.

WHO ARE GOOD CANDIDATES?

The best candidates are men who are relatively young and who do not have severe forms of prostate cancer. Cryotherapy is also commonly used for individuals who have been treated with radiation but whose cancer has recurred. Surgery cannot be performed on most men who have already had radiation treatment, because the radiation destroys anatomical landmarks and causes scar tissue to form; cryotherapy is therefore one of the few options available. In order for it to be effective, the cancer must be confined to the prostate; men with advanced cancers are not candidates. Men whose prostate weighs more than approximately 40 gms are also not appropriate candidates unless the prostate can first be downsized with hormone therapy.

THE PROCEDURE

The procedure is carried out in a hospital, and the patient usually remains overnight. It is performed under local (spinal or epidural) or general anesthesia, with techniques similar to those used in implanting seeds in radiation seed therapy. Long needles are inserted into the prostate through the perineum. A freezing substance (liquid nitrogen was utilized in the past, but argon gas is now used) is inserted through the needles and the prostate is frozen into what is memorably referred to as an ice ball. An ultrasound probe is inserted into the rectum so that the urologist can carefully place the needles and ensure that tissue outside the prostate is not frozen. Because the urethra runs directly through the prostate, a catheter carrying warm, circulating water is inserted through it so that the urethra will not also be frozen. Following the procedure, a urinary catheter is left in place for approximately two weeks, during which time most men do not go back to work.

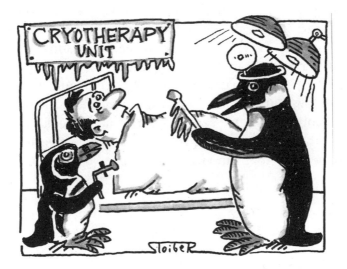

COMPLICATIONS

The complications of cryotherapy are fewer now than in the past. The most dangerous possibility is freezing the wall of the rectum, which is immediately behind the prostate, thereby creating a fistula (hole) between the bladder and the rectum. This complication is very serious, even life-threatening, and the wall must be surgically re-paired. In the past, it occurred in 2 percent of cases but today is much less common.

Urinary retention and long-term incontinence also used to be common, occurring in up to two thirds of cases, but more recent studies have reported an incontinence rate of less than 10 percent.

The most frequent complication is impotence, since it is virtu-ally impossible to freeze the prostate without freezing the adjacent nerves, arteries, and veins running to the penis. One study reported an impotence rate of 87 percent among men who had been potent prior to cryotherapy. As one review summarizes the data, "Cryo-therapy is associated with higher rates of impotence than are most other localized treatment alternatives."[1]

OUTCOME

The long-term outcome of cryotherapy is not yet known, for the technology is still evolving. In one analysis, the cancer recurrence rate two years after treatment, as measured by rising PSA, was 40 per-cent for low-risk, 55 percent for intermediate-risk, and 64 percent for high-risk cancers. In another study, the recurrence rates at seven years were reported to be 39 percent, 32 percent, and 39 percent for men with low-, intermediate-, and high-risk cancers.[2] A special con-cern in cryotherapy is that cancer cells that lie immediately adjacent to the urethra, which is being warmed during the freezing process, may not become frozen and will thus survive.

7

Alternative and
Experimental Therapies

Alternative therapies for medical disorders have become increasingly popular in the United States, with 42 percent of adults reporting having used one or more.[1] The increasing popularity of alternative therapies has been fueled in part by rapid distribution of information on the Internet and in part by dissatisfaction with an increasingly dysfunctional traditional medical care system. Men with prostate cancer are especially susceptible to claims made for alternative therapies, since existing treatments produce a plethora of unfortunate complications.

Alternative medicine covers a broad spectrum of therapies, ranging from special diets, vitamin and mineral supplements, and herbal therapies to hyperthermia, ultrasound, light therapy, gene therapy, magnets, acupuncture, moxibustion, yoga, massage therapy, relaxation exercises, and prayer. There is some evidence that specific dietary factors may be useful in preventing or slowing the growth of prostate cancer; these factors, along with vitamins and minerals, are discussed in Chapter 13. The present chapter will focus on herbal therapies as well as other experimental therapies being studied for the possible treatment of newly diagnosed prostate cancer. Drugs and other experimental treatments for recurrent prostate cancer are examined in Chapter 11.

HERBAL THERAPIES

Herbs are seed plants whose stems wither after each growing season. Herbal therapies are especially attractive to men with prostate cancer, in that they are widely used in China, where the incidence of prostate cancer is very low. Many men assume, therefore, that some cause-and-effect relationship must exist. Herbs are generally considered to be natural, pure, and safe, although this is not always the case. Advocates point out that a quarter of all existing medications, including digitalis and morphine, are derived from plants. Herbal therapies are also popular because the ingredients are available in health food stores and on the Internet without a prescription. Many consumers do not realize that as long as the product is not advertised to treat a specific disease, essentially no regulation or testing of the compounds takes place.

The number of men with prostate cancer who use herbal therapies is impressive, ranging from 10 to 22 percent in various surveys. A study of 238 men treated by surgery or radiation for prostate cancer in Charlottesville, Virginia, reported that 12 percent were also using herbs, and a questionnaire returned by 1,099 men being treated at six major urology treatment centers in the United States revealed that 16 percent were using herbal therapy. Studies of men being screened for prostate cancer show a high utilization of herbal therapies as well, ranging from 21 percent in Denver to 29 percent in Toronto.[2]

The herb that is most popular among men with prostate cancer is saw palmetto, an extract of the dwarf palm that grows in the southeastern United States. It is said that Native Americans used its berries for urinary problems. Extracts of the berries are prepared in a variety of ways and contain a mixture of fatty acids, sterols, flavonoids, and other compounds. The composition of saw palmetto preparations may vary, since its manufacture has not been standardized.

Saw palmetto is thought to have some ability to block testosterone. Tested widely in men with benign prostatic hypertrophy (BPH), it has been found to increase urine flow, decrease urinary obstruction, and decrease the number of times the individual has to get up at night.[3] In one study, saw palmetto was as effective as finasteride

(Proscar), which is widely used to treat BPH; in another study, however, saw palmetto was only one third as effective.

Saw palmetto has not been demonstrated to have any effect on cancer cells but may provide small symptomatic relief by increasing urine flow. Nevertheless, it is widely used for prostate cancer; two studies in Canada reported that 12 and 20 percent of patients were taking saw palmetto, and a study of six American treatment centers reported 16 percent. Saw palmetto is also popular among men who fear getting prostate cancer; in one study 15 percent of brothers of men with prostate cancer were using it.[4]

Several studies of alternative therapies have noted that men who are relatively young and those who have more education, more money, and more advanced prostate cancers than others are more likely to use these therapies. A study in San Francisco comparing the use of alternative therapies by ethnic group found that herbal remedies were used almost equally by white (14 percent), Hispanic (17 percent), African American (19 percent), and Asian (19 percent) men with prostate cancer.[5] The majority of men using herbs or other alternative therapies do not inform their treating physician—but they should do so, for herbs may interact with other medications.

A major problem in evaluating the effectiveness of herbal therapies for treating prostate cancer is that most men do not take just one herb. Many who take saw palmetto, for example, also take pygeum, which comes from the bark of a tree native to Africa, where it has traditionally been used to treat urinary problems. Evaluation becomes even more difficult when men are using combinations of herbs, such as rasagenthi lehyam, a traditional Indian treatment for cancer that contains "38 different botanicals . . . and 8 inorganic compounds, all prepared into a paste in a palm sugar and hen's egg base."[6]

Men who use herbal therapy are likely to be simultaneously using other forms of alternative medicine. Shark cartilage is an example, intermittently used for many years in cancer patients with the mistaken belief that sharks do not get cancer. In a study in the United States, 8 percent of men with prostate cancer were taking shark cartilage, while in a Canadian study, 24 percent were using it. One study of shark cartilage in men with prostate cancer reported that it had no effect; other studies are currently under way, funded by the National

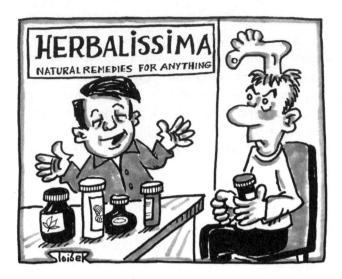

"Well, yes, some of them *do* have side effects."

A Novel Treatment

One of my favorite examples of a patient's strategy comes from a man I know who also has prostate cancer: Instead of imagining his good cells attacking his bad cells, he goes to Europe from time to time and imposes Continental images on his bad cells. He reminds me that in an earlier, more holistic age, doctors used to advise sick people to go abroad for their health.

—Anatole Broyard, *Intoxicated by My Illness*

Center for Complementary Medicine under the National Institutes of Health.[7]

Alternative therapies may, of course, have side effects. For saw palmetto, these include headache, gastrointestinal distress, and increased blood pressure. Other herbal products have been reported to have serious complications in some individuals, including liver fail-ure from kava kava, hepatitis from jin bu huan, and seizures from yohimbe. The risk of such complications is increased by the fact that there is virtually no regulation of the manufacturing or content of these preparations.

PC-SPES: A CAUTIONARY TALE

The most popular herbal treatment for prostate cancer has been PC-SPES, the name being an abbreviation of prostate cancer and the Latin word for "hope." It was commercially available from 1996 until 2002, when its manufacturer, BotanicLab in Brea, California, abruptly shut down. At the time, it was estimated that approximately ten thousand men with prostate cancer were taking PC-SPES and a bottle of sixty capsules was selling for $108. The recommended dose ranged from six to twelve capsules per day, depending on the severity of the man's cancer.[8] If all the men had been taking six capsules a day, sales would have totaled $3.2 million each month.

PC-SPES was formulated by Sophie Chen, a Taiwanese immi-grant who trained in chemistry and initially worked at several large drug companies. She also held an adjunct faculty position at New York Medical College. Her principal collaborator was Xuhui "Allan" Wang, an herbalist who claimed that his great-grandfather had been court physician to a Chinese emperor.[9] Chen and Wang formulated PC-SPES as a combination of six Chinese herbs, a Chinese mush-room, and the American herb saw palmetto. These herbs are believed to have mild estrogenic activity, thus suppressing testosterone. To-gether with Chen's brother, John, they began to manufacture and sell their new formulation. They advertised it as merely being useful for "prostate health," not specifically for cancer or any disease condi-tion, thus avoiding all regulations that require testing for safety and efficacy.

The formulation was an immediate success. Men with prostate cancer noted a rapid decrease in their PSA, and word spread quickly through the Internet and prostate cancer survivor groups. In 1999 *The Herbal Remedy for Prostate Cancer* was published by James Lewis, a Ph.D. in education administration who himself had prostate cancer. It extolled PC-SPES and acknowledged that Sophie Chen had "read the entire manuscript and offered her suggestions which provide accurate assessment of its contents."[10]

By 1999, prostate cancer researchers had begun testing PC-SPES and reporting that it did indeed lower the PSA and shrink the prostate. Michael Milken's Prostate Cancer Foundation gave Chen a grant of $150,000 and provided an additional $500,000 for researchers to test it. The National Center for Complementary and Alternative Medicine, part of the National Institutes of Health, also provided funds. Some of the researchers who were involved in testing PC-SPES were, like Sophie Chen, on the faculty of New York Medical College and from her received "small amounts of company stock."[11]

From the earliest use of PC-SPES, certain side effects were noted. Most prominent was breast enlargement, which was "nearly universal"; in some cases breasts grew so large that men "had to have them surgically removed." Also noted were blood clots in the leg— thromboembolism—which "occurred in approximately 5 percent of patients." Several people, including some of the researchers who were testing PC-SPES, noted the similarity of its side effects to those of diethylstilbestrol (DES), an estrogen compound that effectively suppresses testosterone but that has serious side effects, including thromboembolism. In 2001 an additional side effect of PC-SPES was noted when several men who were taking it began to bleed mysteriously. In one case, reported in a medical journal, a man had "turned up in an emergency room in Idaho bleeding from every orifice, and the hospital had barely saved him."[12]

The denouement of the PC-SPES tale was provided not by the National Institutes of Health or the Food and Drug Administration, but rather by a Connecticut housewife.[13] Her husband had been taking PC-SPES with effective lowering of his PSA until 2001, when the formulation suddenly stopped working. She decided to have various lots of PC-SPES tested for adulteration, and the tests came back positive: the lots of PC-SPES that had been effective had been adulterated with DES, and the lots that were no longer effective did not contain DES. She posted the information on the Internet, and it was quickly confirmed by other laboratories.

In January 2002, the state of California opened an investigation, and it was shown that PC-SPES had been adulterated with DES since its earliest manufacture in 1996. It was also found to be adulterated

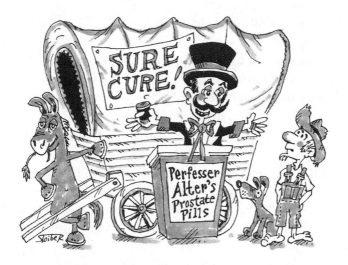

with indomethacin, an anti-inflammatory drug, and warfarin, an anticlotting drug presumably added to try to counteract the DES-caused thromboembolism. In a further investigation by California officials, "the state found adulteration with some pharmaceutical agent in every BotanicLab product that it could test."[14]

BotanicLab as a company pleaded no contest to a felony charge and shut down. Sophie Chen and her brother pleaded no contest to misdemeanor charges, were fined nearly $500,000, and were barred from the dietary supplement business in California. Ms. Chen denied any wrongdoing: "I am just a scientist," she said. "I am only trying to find a cure for cancer."[15]

EXPERIMENTAL TREATMENTS

A variety of alternative therapies for the primary treatment of prostate cancer are in the experimental stages. One such therapy is *hyperthermia*, in which the prostate gland is warmed; this treatment is thought to improve the effectiveness of radiation therapy. The warming may be done by inserting small tubes (interstitial radiofrequency) or small seeds (thermoseeds) directly into the prostate.

An alternative form of hyperthermia is high-intensity focused ultrasound (HIFU), which is being used in Europe and Canada. A probe is inserted into the rectum and, over a period of several hours, sends out ultrasound heat waves that destroy the cancer cells. The main drawback of all forms of hyperthermia is the danger of heat damage to the rectum, urethra, and other adjacent tissue. Whether such treatment will result in fewer complications or better outcomes remains to be ascertained.

A form of *light therapy* is also being studied. A chemical derived from plant chlorophyll is injected intravenously. A laser light source is then beamed into the prostate, causing the chemical to destroy the cancer cells.

Gene therapy is being developed to treat both primary and recurrent prostate cancers. A virus injected into the body goes to the cancer cells, where it delivers a specific gene. This gene makes the cancer cells more susceptible to drugs, which are then administered to the patient.

In addition, various *drugs* are being examined for possible use against prostate cancer. Included are drugs that directly attack cancer cells, drugs that make the cancer cells more susceptible to other forms of treatment, and drugs that cut off the blood supply to the cancer. Most experimental drugs are being developed for recurrent prostate cancer, but a few are directed at primary prostate cancers.

8

Treatment Decisions

Thomas Stamey, a prostate cancer researcher at Stanford University, wrote that when people are "faced with a serious illness beyond their comprehension, [each of us] becomes childlike, afraid, and looking for someone to tell us what to do."[1] In the case of prostate cancer, men are frequently advised by different physicians to do entirely different things and then told: "But in the end, it is up to you to decide." There is probably no other major disease in which the burden of treatment decisions is placed so fully on the shoulders of the patients.

In addition to having to make the treatment decisions, men are warned that these decisions must be made in a timely manner. Some studies have shown that delays in initiating treatment, especially for men with advanced stages of cancer, increase the chances of cancer recurrence. Judd Moul, a prostate cancer specialist at Duke University, counsels: "I have a referral academic practice in which a lot of patients are getting second and third opinions. Some of these patients float from one doctor to another seeking the magic answer. . . . There are a lot of men who become well informed, but this can sometimes lead to paralysis."[2]

This chapter will summarize ten factors that should be considered when choosing a treatment for prostate cancer, and will spell out the advantages and disadvantages of the major treatment options. Before we commence this discussion, however, we need to address the question that crosses every man's mind after being diagnosed with prostate cancer: What will happen if I do nothing?

WATCHFUL WAITING

Prostate cancers are, in general, among the slowest-growing human cancers. Since they usually occur in men who are middle-aged or older, the question arises whether the cancer will kill you before you die from something else.

Several studies have examined the natural course of prostate cancer in men who were not treated. Most were carried out in Scandinavian countries, where medical follow-up is excellent and where it is customary to treat prostate cancer much more conservatively than in the United States. In most European countries, in fact, watchful waiting has been a common approach to prostate cancer, although this tradition is gradually changing, especially in Germany, where radiation treatment has become increasingly popular. In countries with waiting lists for elective surgery, such as England and Canada, a period of watchful waiting is often administratively necessary.

The Scandinavian study that has followed men longest was carried out in Örebro County, Sweden. There, between 1977 and 1984, 223 men were diagnosed with prostate cancer. Their average age was 72, their cancers were all thought to be localized to the prostate, and the cell type was poorly differentiated (that is, more malignant) in only nine cases; this classification was prior to widespread utilization of the Gleason grading system or availability of the PSA. The men therefore fell into the category of having prostate cancers for which watchful waiting is considered a reasonable option. They were closely followed for an average of twenty-one years, by which time 91 percent of them had died.[3]

The percentages of living men whose prostate cancers spread beyond the capsule during five-year follow-up periods were as follows: five years, 32 percent; ten years, 47 percent; fifteen years, 55 percent; and twenty years, 64 percent. A total of 16 percent of the men died from prostate cancer, but in men who were aged 70 or younger at the time of diagnosis, the prostate cancer death rate was 22 percent.

The most surprising finding was that the spread of the cancer and the cancer-related deaths were relatively constant for the first fifteen years after diagnosis but then increased sharply. As summarized by the researchers: "An approximately 3-fold higher rate was found both for progression and death during follow-up beyond 15 years. . . . If such patients are in their 60s or younger, disease progression that occurs after 15 or more years may be a real concern, arguing for early local treatment with a curative intent."[4]

In another Swedish study, 695 men diagnosed with prostate cancer between 1989 and 1999 were randomly assigned to either watchful waiting (348 men) or prostate surgery (347 men). The average age of men in both groups was 65. In the watchful waiting group, 74 percent of the cancers were palpable but had no known spread, and 30 percent had Gleason scores of 7 or higher. At an average follow-up of 6.1 years after diagnosis, among the men being followed by watchful waiting the cancer had spread outside the prostate in 31 percent of cases, had spread to distant organs in 16 percent, and had killed 9 percent of the men. The comparable rates for men treated by surgery were 12, 10, and 5 percent, respectively.[5]

The mortality rates in these Swedish studies for men who were not treated for their cancers are comparable to rates reported in earlier research. A summary of six studies calculated that 13 percent of men with Gleason scores of 7 or lower who were not treated had died from prostate cancer by ten years after diagnosis. For men with Gleason scores of 8 or higher, the death rate was 66 percent.[6]

The most useful American study of watchful waiting has been the Connecticut study of 767 men who were aged 55 to 74 at the time their prostate cancer was diagnosed. All elected watchful waiting and were followed for twenty years, by which time 96 percent had died. The men's Gleason scores were highly predictive of their likelihood of dying from prostate cancer: men with a Gleason score of 5 or less had a 10 percent chance of dying from their prostate cancer; Gleason score 6, a 27 percent chance; Gleason score 7, a 51 percent chance; and Gleason score 8 to 10, a 66 percent chance.

The likelihood of dying from prostate cancer, of course, varied widely by the age of the men at the time of diagnosis; that is, men who were older were more likely to die from other causes before their cancer could kill them. For example, among men with a Gleason score of 7, 73 percent who were 64 or younger at the time of initial diagnosis died from prostate cancer, but among men 65 or older, only 37 percent died from prostate cancer. This study, authored by Peter Albertsen and his colleagues at the University of Connecticut, was published in 2005 and should be reviewed by all men who are considering watchful waiting as a treatment option.[7]

The studies cited above assessed the *quantity* of life for men whose prostate cancers were initially not treated. Other researchers have attempted to assess the *quality* of life for such men. In the first Swedish study, for example, after four years of watchful waiting, 21 percent of the men had frequent urinary leakage (with half of them wearing pads), and 45 percent complained of erectile dysfunction. Similarly, a Danish study followed fifty-two men, average age 69, of whom one third had relatively malignant cell types. By approximately three years after beginning watchful waiting, 31 percent had experienced urethral stricture, 31 percent had required a transurethral resection of the prostate for urinary symptoms, 21 percent were using pads because of symptoms of incontinence, 44 percent had been treated with hormones, 8 percent had required radiation treatment for metastases, 77 percent had impaired erections, and 12 percent were impotent. On the other hand, an American study of 310 men, average age 75, reported some cancer-related decrease in sexual function but no increase in urinary or bowel complaints five years after the onset of watchful waiting.[8]

Thus, for men with intermediate or severe forms of prostate cancer, it appears that the answer to the question, "What will happen if I do nothing?" is reasonably clear. As summarized by one research group:

> It is likely that with watchful waiting, roughly 30% to 40% of men with Gleason sum 6 cancers and well over 50% of men with Gleason sum 7 cancers will be dead of prostate cancer or suffering from progressing, hormonally refractory metastatic disease within 10 to 15 years if not treated definitively, with some additional time (<5 years) added if a patient has stage T1C [not palpable on rectal exam] disease at diagnosis.

These figures are based on the assumption that men who elect watchful waiting do nothing to decrease the chances of their prostate cancer progressing. A 2005 study of forty-four men on watchful waiting who adopted major lifestyle changes, including a vegan diet, exercise, and stress management, suggested that such changes can significantly slow the progression of the cancer.[9] This study is discussed at greater length in Chapter 13.

Depending on one's perspective, the outcome of watchful waiting can be viewed as a glass either half empty or half full, and men with prostate cancer still regularly choose watchful waiting as a treatment alternative. As noted in *Time* magazine: "Faced with this bewildering array of draconian treatments—and their humiliating side effects—many older men and some younger ones opt for watchful waiting." The number of men choosing this option is, however, decreasing; in 1993–1995, 20 percent of men chose watchful waiting, but in 1999–2001, only 8 percent did so.[10]

The best candidates for watchful waiting are men who are over age 70 and whose cancer is in the early stages; for example, nonpalpable on rectal exam, Gleason score of 5 or less, and PSA of 5 or less. Such cancers are statistically likely to grow slowly. Other reasonable candidates for watchful waiting are elderly men with significant health problems, a life expectancy of less than ten more years, and an early-stage cancer. A study of 1,158 men who chose watchful waiting found that three quarters of them were over age 65 and had a Gleason score of 6 or less.[11] Most men who choose watchful waiting get repeat PSAs and digital rectal exams at least twice a year and repeat biopsies yearly to watch for progression of the cancer.

A disadvantage of watchful waiting is living with uncertainty. You are essentially placing a bet, and if you bet wrong, you may lose the window of opportunity to cure the cancer. As Patrick Walsh observed: "When cancer escapes from the prostate, it doesn't send out a press release announcing the event; it just goes, as silently as it appeared in your body in the first place." One man who bet wrong was Willet Whitmore, chief of urology at Memorial Sloan-Kettering Cancer Center in New York and regarded as one of the nation's prostate cancer experts. When he himself got prostate cancer, he chose watchful waiting, but his cancer progressed. Before he died in 1995, "it was reported that he said he regretted the fact that he had waited too long before actively treating his disease." Ironically, Whitmore is most quoted today for his succinct expression of the dilemma of

Watchful Waiting

Morty is a seventy-four-year-old retired magazine editor whose prostate cancer was diagnosed two years ago. His PSA at diagnosis was 11 ng/mL and it has stayed there, plus or minus a point, for the past year. His DRE [digital rectal exam] is normal, he has no symptoms, and his scans are clean. "After my initial diagnosis, I consulted a slew of urologists and radiation specialists," he says. "They all told me I should get carved or get zapped. But I decided instead just to keep an eye on things. Since then, I've been in good health. I sleep through the night without having to get up to pee. I still enjoy the good life, sexually, emotionally, and in every other way. In fact, my life is even better, because I've become vividly aware of how precious each day is."

—David Bostwick et al., *Prostate Cancer*

prostate cancer treatment: "If cure is necessary, is it possible, and if cure is possible, is it necessary?"[12]

In actual practice, watchful waiting is evolving today into nothing more than delayed treatment for many men. The reason, according to Judd Moul, is that "the men just can't stand to see their PSA values going up. Either the patients, their doctors, or a combination of both together get cold feet." Thus, one study of men who chose watchful waiting reported that 53 percent had abandoned the strategy and sought treatment within two years; other studies too have reported significant dropout rates from watchful waiting.[13]

Additional insight on the effectiveness of watchful waiting as a treatment strategy should come from the large Prostate Cancer Intervention Versus Observation Trial (PIVOT) being run by the federal Department of Veterans Affairs. This trial registered 731 men between 1994 and 2002, and results should be available by 2008.

TEN FACTORS TO CONSIDER

Choosing a treatment for your prostate cancer will be easier if you systematically consider each of the following ten factors:

1. *The severity of your cancer*: As described in Chapter 2, prostate cancers can be divided into four groups on the basis of risk of recurrence and progression:

- *Low risk:* Not palpable on rectal exam (T1) or, if palpable, occupies less than half of one lobe (T2a); Gleason score 6 or below; and PSA less than 10.
- *Intermediate risk:* Palpable and occupies more than half of one lobe (T2b) or is in both lobes (T2c); or Gleason score of 7; or PSA of 10 to 20.
- *High risk:* Cancer has spread beyond the capsule of the prostate but not to the seminal vesicles (T3a); or Gleason score of 8 to 10; or PSA greater than 20.
- *Very high risk:* Cancer has spread to seminal vesicles (T3b) or lymph nodes (N+), or has metastasized to bones or other distant organs (M+).

The severity of the cancer can be further refined by consideration of the number of biopsy cores positive for cancer, the percentage of each core containing cancer, and the velocity with which the PSA has risen. The severity of your cancer should be the single largest determinant of your treatment choice.

2. *Your life expectancy: will treatment extend it?*: How long you are likely to live is the second-most important factor in making a treatment decision. As noted in the accompanying box, treatment decisions for a 50-year-old man who is expected to live an additional twenty-five or more years may be quite different from decisions for a 70-year-old man whose life expectancy is less than fifteen more years. Be aware that these life expectancy projections are averages for the entire American male population, and that many medical and lifestyle factors modify these numbers. For example, studies have

shown that a 40-year-old man will lose 3.1 years of life if he is overweight as measured by body mass index (BMI 25–29) and 5.8 years of
life if he is obese (BMI 30 or more), compared to men of normal
weight. If he is both overweight and a smoker, he will lose 6.7 years,
and if obese and a smoker, he will lose 13.7 years.[14]

*In a review of the studies on cancer recurrence, rates of metastasis, and
deaths attributable to prostate cancer, it seems very likely that active treatment extends the life of most, but not all, men who choose it over watchful
waiting.* At this time, there is no evidence that either surgery or beam
radiation has an advantage over the other in this regard; the lower
death rates reported with surgery appear to occur because surgery is
more likely to be offered to younger men with less serious forms of
cancer. Insufficient information is available to determine whether
seed radiation extends life more readily than the other treatments,
but data so far do not suggest that it does.

3. *Your willingness to live with uncertainty*: Some men are more willing than others to live with uncertainty. Retired General Norman
Schwarzkopf is one who is not willing, as he emphatically explained:
"I'm not a type-B personality who knows I have a cancer growing
inside of me and can live with the knowledge." Not surprisingly,
Schwarzkopf chose surgery as his treatment. He falls into the category
of men who say, "I want the cancer out, preferably by yesterday."[15]

Surgery provides the most information about prostate cancer:
its actual size; the true Gleason score based on the entire cancer;
whether the cancer extends into or beyond the capsule; and whether
it has already spread beyond the margins of resection or to the seminal vesicles or lymph nodes. Equally important is the fact that the
PSA following surgery can be used as a predictor of cancer recurrence.
By contrast, radiation treatment provides no information about the
exact pathologic stage of the cancer, and the postradiation PSA is a
less accurate predictor of recurrence, especially in light of the possibility of a PSA bounce. Hormone treatment may also interfere with
the accuracy of the PSA as a predictor of recurrence. For some men,
having this information is less important, and they are willing to
accept some uncertainty in return for what they perceive to be the
advantages of other forms of treatment.

The problem of uncertainty following prostate cancer treatment

Life Expectancy Table

The following are U.S. life expectancy data based on 2002 mortality statistics and published by the Center for Disease Control and Prevention in 2004. Life expectancies in Canada and Western Europe are approximately one year longer.

	Your life expectancy is age:	
If you are age:	White males	Black males
40	77.4	72.8
45	77.9	73.5
50	78.5	74.6
55	79.3	76.0
60	80.3	77.6
65	81.6	79.6
70	83.3	81.8
75	85.3	84.5
80	87.7	87.5
85	90.7	90.8
90	94.1	94.5

Note: Life expectancies are averages for the entire white and black male population. If you have heart problems, hypertension, high cholesterol, diabetes, other serious illness, or are overweight, a smoker, use alcohol excessively, do not exercise, and/or your parents and grandparents died relatively young, deduct a few years from the life expectancy table. If you have none of these factors, add a few years.

SOURCE: E. Arias, United States Life Tables, 2002, *National Vital Statistics Reports* 53 (2004): 1–6.

was assessed in a study of fear of recurrence in men undergoing surgical, external beam radiation, or seed implant radiation treatment. Prior to treatment, the men in all three groups had approximately the same level of fear. Two years after treatment, the men who had undergone surgery had the least fear of recurrence, and those who had been treated with either beam or seed radiation scored approximately 10 percent higher on the fear assessment scale. These results are similar to the findings of better post-op mental health in men who were treated by surgery, compared to those treated by beam radiation, as described in Chapter 3.[16]

4. *Quantity versus quality of life*: Treatment decisions for prostate cancer often involve deciding between the possibility of living longer but not as well and living well but not as long. For example, watchful waiting for a man with a low-risk cancer promises a relatively satisfactory quality of life at least initially, but a definite possibility that he will not live as long as if he were treated. Conversely, choosing surgery may provide a longer life but one with a high probability of at least partial impotence and other side effects.

5. *Sexual function*: The relative importance of sexual function must be considered when making treatment decisions. For some men, it may be the single most significant factor. It is known that, following treatment for prostate cancer, men are more likely to retain acceptable sexual function if they are younger and if they functioned well prior to treatment. However, for the majority of men, the prognosis is poor; as summarized by one research group, "in reality, most [prostate cancer] survivors experience severe and lasting sexual dysfunction and dissatisfaction."[17] Being diagnosed with prostate cancer is, in fact, less traumatic for men who already have some impotence, as opposed to men who still have active sex lives; the former have less to lose.

For a man whose first priority is to preserve sexual function, none of the choices are attractive. Even watchful waiting carries a long-term risk of increasing sexual dysfunction, either from the expanding tumor or from the hormone or radiation therapy that usually becomes necessary as the cancer progresses. However, men who opt for watchful waiting do preserve their existing sexual function for the immediate future, in contrast to all other treatment options.

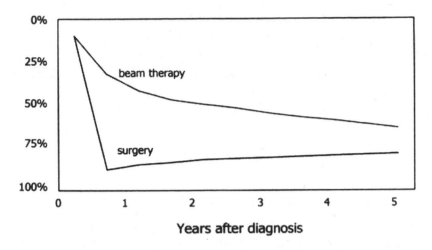

Years after diagnosis

Figure 2. Percentage of Men Reporting Impotence Following Beam Radiation and Surgical Treatment for Prostate Cancer. SOURCE: Data from A. L. Potosky, W. W. Davis, R. M. Hoffman, et al., Five-year outcomes after prostatectomy or radiotherapy for prostate cancer. *Journal of the National Cancer Institute* 96 (2004): 1358–67.

When treatment options other than watchful waiting are compared, radiation treatments preserve sexual function better than surgery for at least the first two years. Fourteen or more studies have compared sexual function after beam radiation and surgery, with the former being found superior every time. Although far fewer studies have compared seed radiation to surgery, they also suggest that seed radiation has an advantage in preserving sexual function for at least the first year following treatment.[18]

For the longer term, the advantage of radiation treatment over surgery in preserving sexual function appears to decrease. The multisite Prostate Cancer Outcomes Study followed 981 surgery and 286 beam radiation patients for five years after treatment. The study defined impotence as an "erection insufficient for intercourse." At two years, 82 percent of men who had had surgery were impotent compared to 50 percent of those who had had beam radiation. At five years, 79 percent of men who had had surgery were impotent compared to 64 percent of those who had had beam radiation.[19] These results, shown in Figure 2, reflect the growing awareness that surgery produces immediate impotence but then gradual improvement that may continue for two years or longer, whereas radiation treatment produces a slow decline in sexual function that may continue for five years or more.

Although seed therapy, based on early reports, was thought to produce less sexual dysfunction than either beam therapy or surgery, this reputation has not held up over time. A study comparing sexual function in 154 men treated with seed therapy and 60 men treated with surgery reported that "sexual function was better with BT [brachytherapy] initially but these differences did not persist at a longer follow-up." In a study that compared all three therapies, men who had undergone seed therapy rated themselves slightly lower on sexual quality of life than men who had undergone either beam therapy or surgery.[20] One reason may be patient satisfaction, which is included in quality-of-life scales. If men choose seed therapy because they expect to retain sexual function but then are disappointed, this dissatisfaction will be reflected in low scores on self-rating questionnaires. Conversely, men who choose surgery expecting to have severe sexual problems sometimes find that the problems are not as bad as they feared, and such men may be comparatively satisfied.

A serious problem in comparing seed therapy with other therapies on any outcome measure is that seed therapy increasingly is accompanied by beam therapy. In 1999 half of all men treated with seed therapy also had beam therapy. Hormone therapy is also being used increasingly often with both seed and beam therapy. In such cases sexual function is invariably lower, usually much lower, than without the second therapy. In a summary of studies of men under age 60, beam therapy alone produced an impotence rate of 50 percent, but beam therapy plus hormones produced a rate of 80 percent. Similarly, seed therapy alone produced an impotence rate of 57 percent, but for seed therapy plus hormones, the rate was 86 percent.[21]

What about Patrick Walsh's claims that "at Johns Hopkins . . . 86 percent of men who undergo surgery are potent"? This frequently cited number is the result of a small study of relatively young men, median age 57, who had early-stage cancers. In almost all cases (89 percent), it was possible to remove the cancer and preserve both nerves. A total of fifty-nine men provided questionnaire data over an eighteen-month period, but only twenty-four men returned all questionnaires; the study has been criticized on other methodological grounds as well.[22] What this study does show is that young men with early-stage prostate cancer retain sexual function when both nerves are preserved; unfortunately, most men with prostate cancer are not this young, and it is sometimes not possible to preserve both nerves because of the size of the tumor.

In summary, if preserving sexual function for the near term is your first priority, your best bet is watchful waiting combined with a lot of luck. Your next-best option is beam or seed radiation alone, which will provide a modest advantage over the surgical option for at least a year or two, although not necessarily for long periods. With surgery, preserving both nerves, if possible, provides a reasonable chance for sexual function, especially for younger men, whereas preserving just one nerve is not auspicious. The worst options for sexual function are surgery with neither nerve preserved, beam and seed radiation together, and any hormone therapy; the incidence of impotence with all of these is very high.

6. *Urinary function*: Problems with urinary function should also be considered when making treatment decisions. For many men, the possibility of being partially or completely incontinent causes greater fear than impotence. Even dripping urine and wearing a pad may have, according to a survey of Medicare patients, "a more significant effect on patients than loss of sexual function."[23]

Multiple comparisons of urinary function following surgery and beam therapy have shown that surgery produces significantly more urinary leakage. In one study, 29 percent of men who had had surgery wore pads to stay dry compared to only 4 percent of men who had had beam therapy. Another study reported that urinary function was worse in men who had had surgery immediately following treatment, but then gradually improved during the first year to almost equal the urinary control of post–beam radiation patients.[24]

Although leaking and other symptoms of urinary incontinence are unusual following radiation treatment, irritative urinary symptoms are not. Such symptoms include frequency, urgency, having to get up several times at night, and trouble starting the urinary stream. Such symptoms appear to be especially common following seed therapy. In one comparative study two years following treatment, men who had had seed therapy complained of irritative urinary symptoms much more often than men who had undergone beam therapy or surgery.[25]

In summary, leaking urine and other symptoms of incontinence are common following prostate surgery, but usually improve over time. Irritative urinary symptoms are more common with radiation treatments, especially seed therapy, and these may persist.

7. *Bowel function*: Prostate cancer treatments may injure the bowel wall, which is located immediately adjacent to the prostate. Comparative studies have consistently shown that this damage is more likely to happen during radiation, especially seed therapy, than during surgery. Bowel symptoms may include diarrhea, urgency, fecal soiling, cramping, and bleeding. In one comparative study of men two years following treatment, 17 percent of those who had been treated with seed therapy assessed bowel difficulties as being a moderate or serious problem, compared to 5 percent of men who had undergone beam therapy and 3 percent of men who had had surgery.[26] Bowel symptoms are worse immediately after radiation, then improve over time but may take as long as two years to stabilize.

8. *Access to a competent doctor*: The accessibility of competent urologists, surgeons, radiologists, and oncologists is another factor to consider when making a treatment decision. If you have access to only one such specialist, or if your health insurer dictates your choice, your treatment decision may be made for you. Relatively few men have the resources to call the physician of their choice and say, "I would like to be scheduled for treatment by you next week and, incidentally, I would like to donate $100,000 to your department research fund." The men who are able to do so always get an appointment.

You should look for a treating physician who is competent and caring, who is interested in you and your problem. He or she should be board certified and not have been subject to any medical disciplinary actions. This information is available from state medical boards and appears on some Internet websites. The best way to find a competent physician is to ask for recommendations from everyone you know who has *any* connection to the medical profession. Widely advertise the fact that you have prostate cancer, so that your friends, and your friends' friends, will help you identify the most competent physicians. One book on prostate cancer cleverly suggests calling the secretaries and nurses in the local department of urology and asking, "Who at your institution would *you* choose to treat your father?"[27] Another source of helpful information is the local prostate cancer support group.

Further, you want a treating physician who performs this procedure on a regular basis. Urologists should be doing at least twenty-five radical prostatectomies per year, and radiation oncologists should be doing at least fifteen seed or beam therapies per year. Multiple studies have shown that high-volume urologists generate significantly fewer immediate and long-term postoperative complications. At the far end of the high-volume spectrum are urologists such as William Catalona at Washington University, Patrick Walsh at Johns Hopkins University, and Peter Scardino at Memorial Sloan-Kettering Cancer Center, who have done, respectively, at least 3,478, 2,494, and 1,000 radical prostatectomies.[28] It is both legitimate and important to ask a potential treating physician approximately how many procedures he or she did last year, and for how many years he or she has been doing them.

It is unfortunately not possible to ask your potential treating physician some of the most crucial questions. These include: How much do you usually drink the night before you treat patients? Are you having an affair with a nurse or technician in the operating room or radiology department that will distract you? Have you done this procedure so often that you are bored and spend most of the time thinking about your golf game or investment portfolio?

For men having surgery, one other question to ask your physician is, Who will assist you in surgery? A radical prostatectomy is a technically difficult procedure that may last four hours or more. The ideal assistant is another board-certified urologist. In university teaching hospitals, the assistant is often a urology or general surgery resident in training who may or may not be competent. If you are having your surgery at a university medical center, you may have to accept that fact.

For men choosing surgery, it is useful to ask your physician about his or her opinion of nerve sparing. This procedure has been practiced for more than twenty years and is known by all board-certified

Select a Urologist, Not a Philosopher

In *Intoxicated by My Illness,* Anatole Broyard said that he would like to discuss his prostate with his urologist "not as a diseased organ but as a philosopher's stone. . . . Is there an Ur-desire, an archeology of passion that antedates or predates the prostate?" You are about as likely to find such a person as you are to find a lawyer who plays Bach's Goldberg Variations while helping you with your will, or a plumber who discusses T. S. Eliot's poetry while fixing your sink. They exist, but they are very rare creatures.

Competent urologists, rather, are highly skilled craftsmen—and that is exactly what you want. They may or may not be good at talking to you, although you should expect them to answer your questions. Medical students who are good at talking often become psychiatrists, and, as a psychiatrist, I can tell you that you certainly do not want one of *us* operating on your prostate.

urologists. Whether or not one or both nerves can be spared depends on the size and position of the cancer, which will not become known until the prostate is being removed. Beware of blanket promises.

Beware also of statistics. If your treating physician overwhelms you with data on how skilled he or she is, or how illustrious the department of urology or radiology is, get another opinion. It is possible to produce advantageous treatment statistics by accepting only easy cases, and some urologists have followed this course. If you are married, it is useful to have your wife join you for interviews with possible treating physicians; women often have better insights than men do. All treating physicians are biased toward their own treatment, but you want to avoid those who are zealots.

9. *Access to a good hospital*: It is vital to have your prostate cancer treated in a hospital that performs many such procedures each year.

These high-volume hospitals have been shown in studies of radical prostatectomy to have fewer surgical deaths and fewer postoperative complications; the same is presumably true for radiation treatment as well. The quality of nursing and anesthesia should also be a matter of serious interest. For men undergoing radiation treatments, ask how modern the equipment is and compare with what you are told at other hospitals; radiation equipment is constantly being improved and upgraded.

The fifty best hospital departments of urology, as published in 2005 by USNews.com, are listed in the box nearby. Be aware that the ranking depends heavily on reputation, which among medical professionals rests largely on research status. Thus, it is possible to have a highly rated hospital that has excellent research but not necessarily excellent clinical care.

Another useful list of hospitals is that of cancer centers designated by the National Cancer Institute. These are hospitals where major cancer research is taking place; it will usually, but not always, include prostate cancer research. As of late 2005, there were sixty-two designated cancer centers, including the well-known Dana-Farber Cancer Institute in Boston, Memorial Sloan-Kettering Cancer Center in New York, M. D. Anderson Cancer Center in Houston, and Fred Hutchinson Cancer Research Center in Seattle. A list of these centers by state can be accessed on the Internet by going to the home page of the National Cancer Institute (www.cancer.gov) and clicking on "Treatment," then on "Treatment Facilities."

Still another list of cancer treatment facilities is the National Comprehensive Cancer Network, nineteen affiliated facilities that are described on the website of the coordinating organizations (www.nccn.org). All of these lists, however, suffer from the same limitation: exemplary cancer research is not necessarily accompanied by exemplary clinical care.

10. *Convenience and cost*: The convenience and cost of prostate cancer treatment options are practical but crucial considerations. Compared to radiation, surgery entails a more prolonged recovery, during which time work and regular activities must be curtailed. The accessibility of the treatment unit should be weighed; having to stay in a hotel in a distant city for several weeks to have beam therapy will be

The Fifty Best Hospitals for Urology in 2005

This ranking is based on a variety of factors, including reputation among medical professionals, ratio of nurses to patients, mortality ratio, and equipment.

1. Johns Hopkins Hospital, Baltimore
2. Cleveland Clinic
3. Mayo Clinic, Rochester, Minn.
4. UCLA Medical Center, Los Angeles
5. New York–Presbyterian Univ. Hosp. of Columbia and Cornell
6. Barnes–Jewish Hospital/Washington University, St. Louis
7. Massachusetts General Hospital, Boston
8. Memorial Sloan-Kettering Cancer Center, New York
9. Duke University Medical Center, Durham, N.C.
10. Stanford Hospital and Clinics, Stanford, Calif.
11. University of Texas, M. D. Anderson Cancer Center, Houston
12. University of California, San Francisco Medical Center
13. Methodist Hospital, Houston
14. University of Michigan Medical Center, Ann Arbor
15. Northwestern Memorial Hospital, Chicago
16. Clarian Health Partners (IU and Methodist Hospitals), Indianapolis
17. Vanderbilt University Medical Center, Nashville
18. Hospital of the University of Pennsylvania, Philadelphia
19. Lahey Clinic, Burlington, Mass.
20. University of Iowa Hospitals and Clinics, Iowa City
21. NYU Medical Center, New York
22. University of Virginia Medical Center, Charlottesville
23. William Beaumont Hospital, Royal Oak, Mich.
24. Parkland Memorial Hospital, Dallas
25. Yale–New Haven Hospital, New Haven, Conn.
26. Shands at the University of Florida, Gainesville

27. University of Miami, Jackson Memorial Hospital
28. Christ Hospital and Medical Center, Oak Lawn, Ill.
29. St. Luke's Medical Center, Milwaukee
30. University of Wisconsin Hospital and Clinics, Madison
31. University of Pittsburgh Medical Center
32. Ohio State University Hospital, Columbus
33. Sentara Norfolk General Hospital, Norfolk, Va.
34. Abbott Northwestern Hospital, Minneapolis
35. University of North Carolina Hospitals, Chapel Hill
36. Rush University Medical Center, Chicago
37. Henry Ford Hospital, Detroit
38. Sarasota Memorial Hospital, Fla.
39. University Hospitals of Cleveland
40. Texas Heart Institute at St. Luke's Episcopal Hospital, Houston
41. University of Colorado Hospital, Denver
42. Brigham and Women's Hospital, Boston
43. University Hospital, Cincinnati
44. Advocate Lutheran General Hospital, Park Ridge, Ill.
45. Lancaster General Hospital, Pa.
46. University Medical Center, Tucson, Ariz.
47. F. G. McGaw Hospital at Loyola University, Maywood, Ill.
48. University of Minnesota Medical Center, Minneapolis
49. Memorial Hermann Hospital, Houston
50. St. Elizabeth Hospital Medical Center, Youngstown, Ohio

SOURCE: Best Hospitals 2005, Urology, USNews.com, http://www.usnews.com (click on "Rankings and Guides," then on "Best Hospitals," then on "Urology").

less pleasant and more expensive than having seed therapy or surgery at a local hospital.

Except for watchful waiting, all treatments for prostate cancer are expensive. An analysis of total costs for the initial workup, treatment, and six months of follow-up in the mid-1990s reported them to be as follows:[29]

Treatment	Total costs
Seed radiation	$15,301
Beam radiation	$15,937
Surgery	$19,019
Seed plus beam radiation	$24,407
Surgery plus beam radiation	$31,329

Since these costs were based on data from 1993 to 1996, the costs today would be still higher.

Ascertaining who will pay the costs of treating your prostate cancer varies from complex to Byzantine. If you are 65 or older, you are covered by Medicare, part A, for the costs of hospitalization; you may also be covered by Medicare, part B, for the costs of the treating physicians. However, you have to pay a deductible and approximately 20 percent of the cost (the copayment), and you have to use physicians who accept Medicare assignment (most do). If you are an armed forces veteran, you may be eligible to use programs at military or Veterans Administration hospitals (the treatment program at Walter Reed Army Hospital in Washington, D.C., for example, is excellent). Or you may be able to use Tricare coverage for most treatment costs by other providers who participate in the Tricare program.

If you have private insurance, such as Blue Cross/Blue Shield or Aetna, coverage for costs varies widely by your specific plan and your location. The insurance plans of large companies usually offer more generous coverage than the plans of small companies. In some plans, you are restricted to using a select list of hospitals and physicians, whereas other plans allow you to choose your own. Virtually all plans pay only a "reasonable and customary fee," which is determined by zip code and varies by region. You will almost certainly

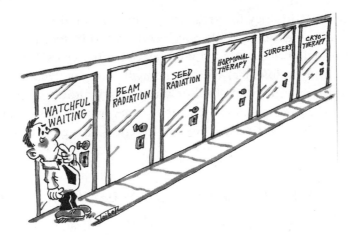

pay a portion of the bill, and the more expensive the physician you select, the higher your portion of the bill is likely to be. Managed-care companies also restrict your options. One study found that Health Maintenance Organizations (HMOs) were more likely to have men treated by radiation than by surgery, since radiation entails lower hospitalization costs.[30]

For men under the age of 65 who do not have health insurance, Medicaid is the best means of coverage. Qualifications differ widely by state. Medicaid coverage is roughly similar to that of Medicare, and you must use physicians who accept Medicaid, which many do not. A useful analysis of payment systems for covering prostate cancer treatment can be found in *Prostate Cancer: A Survivor's Guide,* by Don Kaltenbach and Tim Richards (Seneca House Press, 2003).

Once these ten factors have been considered, many men look for a definitive treatment trial to tell them what to do. Unfortunately, the definitive treatment trial is a myth. Because the treatment of prostate cancer is constantly changing and because prostate cancer progresses so slowly, the information provided by most treatment trials is out of date by the time it becomes available. In my case, I wished that twenty years ago researchers had started a comparison of surgical versus beam radiation treatment so that I would know the long-term outcomes regarding death rate, side effects, and the like. Of course, such a comparison is never going to happen, because the treatment technology for prostate cancer is a moving target. Many comparative treatment trials have been started in recent years, but the results will not be known for fifteen or twenty years. By that time surgical and radiological techniques will have evolved, combinations of treatment will be routinely used, and additional treatment options will be available. And at that time, we will wish that comparative treatment trials had been started now, using the technology of the future.

ADVANTAGES AND DISADVANTAGES OF TREATMENT OPTIONS

In *Seeds of Hope,* Michael Dorso decried the contradictory and confusing advice he found in the medical literature on prostate cancer treatments. Urologists advocated surgery, radiologists advocated radiation treatment, and "cancer specialists who were neither surgeons nor radiation therapists were split between the two treatment modalities." Moreover, a panel of experts in the American Urological Association tried to objectively settle the treatment issues but "found the data inadequate for valid comparisons of treatment. . . . Basically they gave up!" Dorso, himself a physician with prostate cancer, concluded in a note of exasperation: "What's a mother to do?"[31]

That is a very reasonable question. If a physician with prostate cancer has difficulty sorting out the treatment options, how can a layman be expected to do so? And yet that is the message given by most prostate cancer specialists: "In the final analysis, Mr. Smith, the decision is up to you."

In an effort to help men assess the options, the following sections summarize some advantages and disadvantages of each of the major treatment options. These observations should be regarded as general considerations to which there are always exceptions.

Watchful Waiting

Candidates: Men with early-stage cancer (nonpalpable; PSA and Gleason score 5 or less) who are over age 70 or who expect to live less than ten more years. Some men choose this option if short-term preservation of sexual function is paramount.

Chance of cure: Remote.

Convenience: Excellent; a rectal exam, a PSA test, and possibly a biopsy every few months are usually all that is necessary.

Sexual side effects: None unless the cancer progresses.

Urinary side effects: None unless the cancer progresses.

Bowel side effects: None unless the cancer progresses.

Other side effects: None.

Follow-up treatment if needed: PSA is only moderately useful as a marker, since the cancer can spread even with a low PSA. The PSA velocity may be more useful. All treatment options remain open unless the cancer spreads outside the prostate.

Uncertainties: Many; you know you have an untreated cancer growing inside you.

Unknowns: Rate of growth; whether the cancer has spread; precise Gleason score.

Surgery

Candidates: Any man up to approximately age 75 if he is in good health, has a life expectancy of at least ten more years, and there is no evidence of cancer outside the prostate. Many cardiac and other serious medical conditions make men ineligible for surgical treatment.

Chance of cure: Good, if the cancer has not spread beyond the prostate.

Convenience: Highly inconvenient in that it involves major surgery with anesthesia and several weeks of recuperation.

Sexual side effects: Rate of impotence 40 to 90 percent depending on the man's age and whether nerve sparing is possible. Maximum impotence immediately after surgery, then may slowly improve for two years or longer.

Urinary side effects: High rate of incontinence immediately after surgery, then usually improves. Use of pads after two years is 5 to 10 percent. Occasional urinary stricture.

Bowel side effects: Minimal.

Other side effects: Weakness and risk of blood clotting (thrombosis) following surgery.

Follow-up treatment if needed: Beam radiation and hormone therapy commonly used. Seed radiation not possible.

Uncertainties: Less worry than any other treatment. Surgery provides accurate information on the cell type, size, and margins of the tumor and whether the cancer has spread to the lymph nodes, seminal vesicles, and other organs. Post-op PSA is an accurate indicator of recurrence.

Unknowns: The possibility that the cancer has spread beyond the prostate, not detected at surgery.

Beam Radiation Therapy

Candidates: Any man of any age, even if he is not in good health, has a life expectancy of less than ten years, or has cancer that has spread beyond the prostate. Not appropriate for very large prostates unless initially shrunk by hormone therapy, nor for men with chronic bowel disease.

Chance of cure: Good, if cancer has not spread beyond the prostate.

Convenience: Depends on the proximity of the hospital or treatment unit, since it requires daily outpatient treatment five days a week for five to nine weeks. No anesthesia, no surgery, no hospitalization, and no pain. No restriction on activities.

Sexual side effects: Initially minimal, but impotence slowly increases over several years to 40 to 60 percent. Rate higher if combined with seed or hormone therapy.

Urinary side effects: Incontinence rate lower than for surgery but still a small risk. Irritative urinary symptoms and bleeding may be severe and persistent.

Bowel side effects: Frequency, urgency, cramping, and bleeding occur in 10 to 20 percent of cases and may be persistent.

Other side effects: Occasional loss of pubic hair. Fatigue during treatment common. Rectal fistulas now rare.

Follow-up treatment if needed: Surgical treatment difficult because radiation distorts anatomical landmarks and causes scarring of tissues; other options open.

Uncertainties: Provides little information on extent of cancer and possible spread. Posttreatment PSA ambiguous as a predictor of recurrence, especially with PSA bounce.

Unknown: Chances of residual prostate cancer in remaining prostate cells; likelihood of another form of cancer secondary to radiation effects; chances that the cancer has already spread beyond the prostate.

Seed Radiation

Candidates: Men of any age but with a Gleason score 6 or less and a PSA less than 10. Minor surgery required, so may not be appropriate for some men with severe medical conditions. Not suggested for very large prostates unless initially shrunk by hormone therapy, nor for men with chronic bowel disease. Not appropriate for men who have had surgery for BPH.

Chance of cure: Appears favorable so far, but long-term data are not yet available.

Convenience: Very convenient, usually requiring only outpatient surgery with rapid recovery. No restriction of activities except for the first few days.

Sexual side effects: Initially minimal, but impotence slowly increases over several years to 40 to 60 percent. Has the unsupported reputation of causing less sexual dysfunction than beam therapy. Painful orgasm and blood in ejaculate have been reported. Rate of impotence much higher if beam therapy or hormone therapy is used with seed therapy.

Urinary side effects: Incontinence rate lower than surgery but still 5 to 10 percent. Irritative urinary symptoms may be severe and persistent, more so than for beam therapy.

Bowel side effects: Frequency, urgency, cramping, and bleeding occur in 10 to 20 percent of patients and may be persistent.

Other side effects: Men are mildly radioactive for up to two months.

Follow-up treatment if needed: Surgical treatment difficult because radiation distorts anatomical landmarks and causes scarring of tissue; other options open.

Uncertainties: Provides little information on extent of cancer and possible spread. Posttreatment PSA is unclear as a predictor of recurrence, especially with PSA bounce.

Unknowns: Chances of residual prostate cancer in remaining prostate cells; likelihood of another form of cancer secondary to radiation effects; chances that the cancer has already spread beyond the prostate.

Hormone Therapy

Candidates: Any man, even those not in good health or with a life expectancy of less than ten more years. Can be used to shrink large prostates prior to radiation treatment; used with radiation treatment for men with cancers likely to spread (Gleason scores 8 to 10) or that have spread locally, and for cancers that have spread distantly to bones or other organs.

Chances of cure: Remote; hormones slow cancer growth but usually do not kill all the cancer cells.

Convenience: Antiandrogens are taken daily as pills; LHRH agonists are given by intramuscular injections every one, three, or four months.

Sexual side effects: Impotence and loss of libido in almost all cases if given long term; effects occur more slowly with antiandrogens alone.

Urinary side effects: None.

Bowel side effects: None.

Other side effects: Hot flashes; breast tenderness and enlargement; osteoporosis, with possible fractures; fatigue; anemia; weight gain; increased cholesterol; short-term worsening of cancer symptoms (flair) when starting on LHRH agonists.

Follow-up treatment if needed: All options open.

Uncertainties: Hormones interfere with PSA levels, so not useful as a marker for cancer progression.

Unknowns: Rate of growth; whether the cancer is continuing to spread.

Cryotherapy

Candidates: Used mainly as a secondary treatment for men who have had radiation treatment, whose cancer has recurred but not spread beyond the prostate. Not useful for men with large prostates.

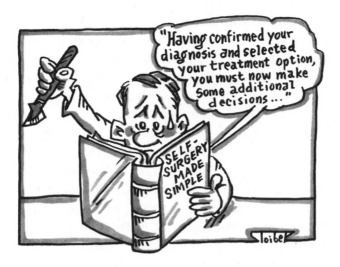

Chances of cure: Insufficient data.

Convenience: Done under anesthesia, usually with overnight hospital stay. Man usually off work for two weeks.

Sexual side effects: Impotence very common, up to 90 percent.

Urinary side effects: Incontinence approximately 10 percent.

Bowel side effects: Low incidence of injury to rectal wall, including fistula, which can be difficult to repair.

Other side effects: None.

Follow-up treatment if needed: Surgical treatment extremely difficult, other options open. Cryotherapy can be repeated multiple times.

Uncertainties: Whether all cancer cells have been killed, especially those close to the urethra.

Unknowns: Long-term effectiveness; chances that the cancer has already spread beyond the prostate.

HOW I MADE MY DECISIONS

My own biggest problem initially was fully comprehending that I had cancer, with its possible implications for my life. I felt mortal in a way that I never had before. I noticed it in little things, like a brief hesitation over whether I should renew a medical journal subscription for one year or three years.

By talking to my wife and medical colleagues, I developed a plan of attack. I read two of the most widely used books on prostate cancer and checked a few websites, but was disappointed with what I found. Much of the information seemed biased toward one treatment or another, and some of the websites were openly commercial. In discussing the cancer with my family and friends, I realized that I had a strong support system already in place.

I next assessed the severity of my cancer. Having a Gleason score of 7 was not advantageous, but the fact that it was 3+4 and not 4+3 was helpful. Three of my nine biopsy cores contained cancer cells, which occupied 20 percent of the core in two cases and 5 percent in the third. Gleason grade 4 cells constituted 40 percent of the cancer cells in one core and 20 percent in the second, and there were no grade 4 cells in the third. The fact that all three positive cores were in the right half of my prostate seemed to confirm the impression of my urologist that the cancer was confined to the right lobe but occupied more than half the lobe; thus, the cancer was probably a stage T2b.

The fact that my PSA was only 3.3 seemed promising. My previous PSA had been 2.0 but had been measured almost four years previously; I was deeply embarrassed to realize that I had gone that long without a PSA test and thus could not assess my PSA velocity over the past year. Overall, my assessment of the severity of the cancer produced a mixed outcome: "intermediate" was the official term, which translated into "it could be worse, but it certainly could be better."

In assessing treatment options, I quickly ruled out watchful waiting and seed radiation therapy as not appropriate for my Gleason 7 cancer. Hormone therapy by itself also seemed inappropriate, since it would not cure the cancer and brought with it serious side effects. That left beam radiation therapy and surgery as the logical options. I calculated my life expectancy to be more than fifteen years. A major factor in my ultimate decision was a distinct unwillingness to live with uncertainty. Surgery for me offered the advantages of finding out the precise severity of the cancer and also being able to use the PSA postoperatively to ascertain possible recurrence.

I thought carefully about the possible side effects of surgery. The odds of urinary incontinence beyond the first few weeks seemed relatively low, and I thought that I could live with pads if necessary.

I did not like the threat of impotence at all, but I had had a long and satisfying sex life and was willing to barter it if necessary for a possible cancer cure and additional years of productive life. Given the apparent size and position of my cancer, I was not optimistic about saving both nerves but was hopeful that one could be saved, thereby providing a reasonable chance of continuing to have a sex life. I discussed the possible outcome extensively with my wife, who was extremely supportive and agreed with my decision. Having been happily married for thirty-seven years seemed a great advantage in this situation.

Once I had decided on surgery, the next questions were "who" and "where." My medical colleagues were extremely helpful in this regard, and I quickly ascertained that there were at least three Washington-area urologists who were highly regarded. One of them, Nicholas Constantinople, was the urologist who had performed my biopsy and whom I liked. I also explored the possibility of going to Johns Hopkins Hospital in Baltimore, where I had close research ties and visited regularly. I had a cordial telephone conversation with Patrick Walsh, who was then chief of urology, and investigated clinical aspects of the hospital. I also ascertained that my medical insurance plan would cover the cost of treatment and that I had abundant sick leave available.

After weighing all the options, I decided to have my surgery done by Dr. Constantinople at Sibley Memorial Hospital, a highly regarded community hospital a mile from my home. A medical colleague on staff there had verified its reputation for excellent anesthesiologists and nurses and a fine radiology department with the latest equipment in case I needed follow-up beam radiation after surgery. I liked the idea that my urologist would be assisted in surgery by one of his board-certified urologist partners, not by a resident in training. In my medical training years, I had performed my first biopsy, appendectomy, and Caesarian section under the watchful eyes of an attending surgeon and understood that such supervisory surgery is necessary. When it came to suturing *my* severed urethra to *my* bladder in a manner that might determine my lifetime urinary continence, however, I opted for proven experience.

In retrospect, I would make the same decisions again, except that I would probably buy more good red wine to help me with the decision making.

9

Your Support System

It is said that being diagnosed with cancer changes a person forever. My internist, who is a personal friend and who discovered my cancer, said exactly that to me. I did not doubt him then, and I certainly do not doubt him now. A cancer diagnosis is one of life's defining moments, a new tint to one's glasses that puts the world in a different light.

Cancer doesn't just change the person, however. It also changes the person's relationships with family members, friends, coworkers, and professional colleagues. It is not only that *you* see the world in a different light but also that *others* see you in a different light. You are still the person they knew before, but you have something added, "the big C," as it is often called. It is not as stigmatizing as the embroidered "A" that Hester Prynne had to wear in Nathaniel Hawthorne's story, as she stood in the public pillory holding her illegitimate child, but it occasionally feels that way.

YOURSELF

The most important part of your support system, by far, is yourself. This is true even if you have been well married for thirty-seven years, have a daughter and son-in-law who are both physicians, and have

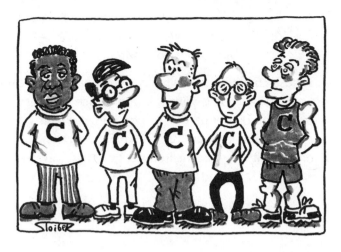

"Sometimes I have a feeling people know we have prostate cancer."

close friends, as I was fortunate to have at the time of my diagnosis. It is equally true if you are living alone, estranged from your family, and have no close friends, as is too often the case. Regardless of your relationships with others, cancer affects your inner self in a way that others cannot see. Every cancer can be said to spread to your soul, even if it never spreads to any other organ.

To utilize your own inner strength in dealing with prostate cancer, men must wrestle with four "i's": the myth of *immortality*, accepting *immodesty*, the fear of *incontinence*, and the fear of *impotence*. Those who successfully confront these demons will find the going much easier. Those who fail to do so will be plagued by a fifth "i"— *indecision*. They will also be prone to denial and depression. The latter can become a major problem; a study in Florida reported that suicide among men with prostate cancer was four times more common than among all men in their same age group.[1]

The myth of one's own immortality confronts everyone with cancer, not just men with prostate cancer. It is the realization, usually for the first time, that "mortal" has two meanings: a human being, and one who is subject to death. Before being diagnosed with cancer or another potentially fatal disease, we secretly believe that we are amaranths; the diagnosis of cancer rapidly wilts our petals, and death becomes real. As Richard Handy noted after being diagnosed

My Closest Possession

The diagnosis changes everything. . . . Now cancer will be my closest possession, going with me from office to house, to conferences and dinner parties, as I go myself. I have got to get used to having it always here. I have got to think about what influence it may assume in time, not only over me but on my family, friends, and work.

—Cornelius Ryan, *A Private Battle*

with prostate cancer, "Cancer permanently severed me from the long youthful tie of emotionally believing myself to be immortal—despite all of aging's warnings that I wasn't."[2]

I was surprised by some of my own thoughts in reaction to the reality of dying. Understandably, I wondered whether I would see my two grandchildren graduate from college, and whether my professional research would come to full fruition. But I also wondered about more mundane things, like whether I would live to see the Red Sox beat the Yankees and win a World Series. Miraculously, five months later it happened! Then I said to myself, but what about the Chicago Cubs?

Confronted with the reality of death, many men react initially with anger and self-pity. Cornelius Ryan, a successful writer, was diagnosed with advanced prostate cancer at age 50 and reflected such thoughts:

I feel such a terrible sense of injustice. What did I do to deserve this? Yet, that's just the kind of question I've got to eliminate from my mind. I do not exactly trust my ability to maintain objectivity publicly unless I can release the body quakes and shocks in private. And how can you make people who haven't got cancer understand what's happened to you without having to endure their pity as well? I'm damned if I want pity. Self-pity is bad enough.

Anger is especially prominent in individuals who feel unfulfilled professionally and those who have deferred activities they enjoy until

> ### Irony
>
> Now at last I understand the conditional nature of the human condition. Yet, unlike Kierkegaard and Sartre, I'm not interested in the irony of my position. Cancer cures you of irony. Perhaps my irony was all in my prostate.
>
> —Anatole Broyard, *Intoxicated by My Illness*

their hoped-for golden years of retirement. Although anger is a natural reaction to being diagnosed with cancer, it serves no useful purpose. As one man noted, such anger is "like a catheter inserted in your soul, draining your spirit."[3]

The myth of one's immortality can be resolved in a variety of ways. The most common is through religious belief, a conviction that your cancer is part of a divine plan and that dying is merely a way station to a life hereafter. This approach is well illustrated by Chuck and Martha Wheeler in their book *Affirming the Darkness.* Chuck was diagnosed with advanced prostate cancer at age 65. He lived eight painful, complication-filled years but mastered his fear of death through his religious belief.

Another approach is through intellectual acceptance. In the words of Francis Bacon, "It is as natural to die as to be born." In this regard, it is helpful to have had an acquaintance with death. For individuals whose sole experience with death has been that of a beloved pet or an elderly grandparent, the initial confrontation with their own potential demise is likely to be deeply troubling. Some of us, by contrast, have met death early and often. I lost my father when I was a child, my own child and two very close friends in my early twenties, and a few years later my mother and a sister to cancer. As a young physician, I cared for people who were dying, pronounced people dead, and had the task of informing their relatives. Death never becomes one's friend, but experience can at least make it an acquaintance. As such, it seems less demonic.

The second challenge in strengthening the self is to accept immodesty as a reality. Most men are reluctant even to talk about their genitals and their sex life, to say nothing of displaying their genitals to the world. Having prostate cancer, however, makes this necessary. Physicians probe your rectum with their fingers. The fingers are replaced by instruments and what sounds like a staple gun during your biopsy. And then, during treatment, you get to show your genitals to a variety of technicians, nurses, and physicians. As Richard Handy described it: "My penis and anus, the parts of my body I had most carefully closeted, were now open to inspection by anyone dressed in white who wanted to look at them. They were no longer protected by modesty or guarded by will."[4]

For individuals who have been taught that their genitals are dirty and disgusting, this openness can be a problem. Cornelius Ryan experienced such feelings:

> I was embarrassed by what was happening in a way that's difficult to describe. Perhaps being fastidious about that part of the body, one can't help having a feeling that what was happening was repulsive. I felt that I was dirty. I didn't put my underwear in with the house laundry and I couldn't let Katie wash it. It was something I had to do myself. I didn't want anyone, not even Katie, to witness the evidence of my disgust and humiliation.[5]

The reality, of course, is that medical personnel who are dealing with urological patients see genitals all day, every day. You may believe that yours are special because they belong to you, but others will probably not give your genitals more than a passing glance. If you can accept immodesty as your new way of life, the diagnosis and treatment of your prostate cancer will go infinitely more smoothly. Personally, I found it comforting to imagine myself on a nude beach in California where, after the first few minutes, nobody paid much attention to anybody else.

The third and fourth issues that must be confronted to strengthen oneself in dealing with prostate cancer are the two principal complications of treatment: urinary incontinence and impotence. Both may vary from being minor annoyances to being major problems, depending on one's age, choice of treatment, and luck of the draw. And for both, treatments are available, as will be discussed in Chapter 10.

Urinary incontinence is essentially a plumbing problem and should be regarded as such, similar to having a chronically leaky bathroom faucet. Urine is, in most individuals, similar to sterile water. It is not harmful in any way, and in disasters, such as being stranded on a mountain ledge or an isolated island, many have saved their lives by drinking their own urine.

Although men may be deeply embarrassed to leak urine, those closest to them may be less concerned. Desiree Howe, in writing about her husband's post-prostatectomy incontinence, put the problem in proper perspective:

> Continence was way down the list of characteristics I sought in a man. Integrity, compassion, intelligence, humor, courage, etc., were Dick's qualities, all of which were high on my check-list. It didn't hurt that he was very good looking, too. Solutions for incontinence were available, but cures for poor character are more difficult, if not impossible, to find.[6]

Singer-actor Robert Goulet also displayed a remarkable attitude toward his urinary incontinence. Three weeks after having surgery for prostate cancer, he rejoined the cast of *Camelot,* wearing a diaper under his pants. He later recounted on national television what happened on stage during the first show:

> Well, right in the middle of the show, there's a scene where I'm all alone on center stage, standing on top of a small hill, spotlit, with my legs spread, singing my heart out. I hit one particular high note, and, sure enough, my bladder gushed away. I could feel my eyes widening. I didn't think the audience could actually tell what had happened, but after the show, I asked Patricia Keyes, my costar, if she noticed anything, well, strange, during that song. And she said, "There was nothing obvious, Robert, but when I saw that twinkle in your eye, I knew it meant a tinkle down your thigh."[7]

Compared to incontinence, the problem of impotence is both more common and more difficult to deal with. Erections define being a man from adolescence on, and for many men the inability to have erections suggests that they are no longer men. The problem is especially troublesome for younger men, for men who believe they have not had their share of sexual adventure and plan to do so in the future, and for older men who have just married a 30-something wife.

> ### Talking About It
>
> There was also another fear: that somehow my incontinence would be obvious to people. Peculiar to fear this, Margaret said, considering my tendency to talk too much about it, to bring people's attention to it when there was no need to. It is an occupational hazard of cancer, whatever form it takes, this need to talk about it.
>
> —Michael Korda, *Man to Man*

It is factors such as these that incline some men toward watchful waiting, deferring definitive treatment of their prostate cancer while they continue to have an active sex life. Against this must be weighed the risk of having the cancer spread. Rudy Giuliani, then mayor of New York City, summarized this dilemma in a national television interview: "The first thing you've got to come to terms with is if you don't live, you can't have sexual function."[8] Similarly, Leon Prochnik titled his book about prostate cancer *You Can't Make Love if You're Dead.*

Personally, I regarded the possibility of impotence following prostate cancer treatment as appalling. However, I regarded the possibility of death from prostate cancer itself as more appalling. I also took great satisfaction in knowing that I had had a full and satisfying sex life and realized that I had stored up sufficient memories to last for the rest of my life. If necessary, I could relive and replay them endlessly, slowly turning them over in my mind, like Marcel Proust's petits madeleines in his *Remembrance of Things Past.*

FAMILY AND FRIENDS

For a man who is married or living with a partner in a long-term relationship, the other person will be affected by the prostate cancer almost as much as he will. As one wife phrased it: "He got the diagnosis, but we both have prostate cancer."[9] It is therefore imperative to include the other person from the beginning in discussions of your cancer; men who initially keep the news from their partner invariably find they have made a mistake.

Wives and partners can be extremely supportive and helpful in such situations. They can collect and organize information on treatment options, especially given the plethora of books and websites available. Many men have found it useful to have their wives accompany them to meetings with their urologists, since it is difficult to remember everything they are being told. Women sometimes ask questions men are reluctant to raise because of embarrassment or timidity.

Another task partners can help with is organizing and paying the medical bills. The administrative complexity of the American medical care system is beyond belief. The *New York Times* noted that when you become a patient in the United States, "you enter a world of paperwork so surreal that it belongs in one of Kafka's tales of the triumph of faceless bureaucracy."[10] Even though I am a physician and should theoretically understand the medical payment system, nobody really can do so. I wanted to focus on my treatment and recovery, so my wife took full responsibility for sorting out what had been, or needed to be, paid by Medicare, Tricare, Blue Cross, or us. Despite the fact that she is an economist, the task proved to be extremely complex and confusing; the bills took more than a year to sort out. I concluded that having the surgery was, in fact, easier than sorting out the payments.

The ultimate measure of wives' value in helping husbands was demonstrated by a 1996 study showing that married men with prostate cancer, on average, live 40 percent longer than single men; the statistics on divorced men fell between the two.[11] The importance of a wife as a support system is also illustrated by personal accounts, such as Chuck and Martha Wheeler's *Affirming the Darkness* and Michael Korda's *Man to Man* (see Appendix B).

In a stable marriage, confronting prostate cancer together can strengthen the husband-wife bond. My own wife was, and continues to be, a wonderful help in getting through my prostate cancer experience. In thirty-seven years of marriage we had shared many challenges, including raising children and living for a year in a remote Arctic village. Prior to marrying, we had each worked for two years in

---

A Wife's Anger

I was angry that Charles had not gone in for treatment earlier; angry because he refused to get a second opinion, and angry that through all of his suffering, he didn't seem serious enough about getting to the root of his problem. I was angry that the first physician didn't give him a more thorough examination, and that he didn't demand more tests after Charles didn't improve from the medication he prescribed.

—Valerie Williams in Charles Williams and Vernon Williams,
That Black Men Might Live

---

the Peace Corps in Africa. We viewed my prostate cancer as an unwelcome but novel challenge, one that we would confront and manage together. If I had had to do so, I could have managed it as a single man, but having a supportive partner made the experience infinitely easier.

Of course, not all marriages are stable, and in such situations prostate cancer, like any other serious illness, can exacerbate marital problems. The wife may blame her husband for not having gotten a regular medical checkup or PSA test. She may resent the loss of income made necessary by her husband's illness, or having to take care of him. She may feel cheated out of her quiet retirement years; as one wife put it, "Both of us are retired and we had hopes . . . of doing all the things we planned." Even in solid marriages prostate cancer tends to divide couples. As another wife put it: "The doctor's findings had already begun to make a difference. Cancer had separated us. In spite of physical closeness a barrier, invisible but everlasting, had come between us."[12]

Impotence inevitably affects wives, which is another reason for involving them in treatment decisions. The assumption is generally made that a wife views her husband's impotence as a great loss. Usually this is true, especially for younger wives, but since prostate cancer occurs most commonly after the age of 60, some wives in that age group have a diminished interest in sex and therefore may not view their husband's impotence as a major loss. In a study comparing husbands and wives on their degree of concern about impotence and urinary incontinence following prostate surgery, wives were substantially less concerned than husbands.[13]

All of the foregoing, and most books on prostate cancer, assume that the man's partner is a woman. Gay men, of course, have men as partners, who are equally as affected by the prostate cancer as wives or girlfriends are. In one of the few pieces written about prostate cancer in gay men, Thomas Blank at the University of Connecticut discussed differences in the two types of situation. For example, possible rectal side effects may be more serious than urinary side effects for some gay men, inclining them away from radiation as a treatment.[14] *A Gay Man's Guide to Prostate Cancer,* edited by Gerald Perlman and Jack Drescher, includes much useful information.

Other family members and friends are also integral parts of a man's support network. I was fortunate in having friends who are medical professionals, several of whom were helpful in obtaining information about urologists, anesthesiologists, the advantages and disadvantages of various hospitals, and other factors that went into my decision making. Their personal support was extremely important and stands out in my mind as one of the high points of the period preceding and following my surgery.

In deciding how to handle the news of prostate cancer with other family members and close friends, be aware that their reaction is likely to depend on your definition of the situation. If you seem to have the problem under control and can discuss it in a calm, factual way, they will usually accept it. If, on the other hand, you are unable to discuss it at all, or break down each time you do, their reaction may not be helpful. One man wrote that what a man with prostate cancer wants most from friends is not merely love but also "an appreciative grasp of his situation, what is known now in the literature of illness as 'empathetic witnessing.' "[15]

Of course, some family members and friends have multiple problems of their own and may not be able to react appropriately. Cornelius Ryan described such a reaction when he told a couple, previously close friends, that he had prostate cancer:

I know I didn't imagine the sudden change in atmosphere. I sensed that Katie noticed it as well. It was as though I had, in an instant, become a totally different person in our friends' view. I felt as though I had committed some unpardonable gaffe, some serious breach of social etiquette. They averted their eyes. There was silence and then they embarrassedly expressed regrets.

Michael Korda also recorded the reactions of friends to his news. "The more people were obsessed with their own health and spiritual well-being, I discovered, the more likely they were to be unable to deal with the subject of cancer." Richard Handy's older brother "never called or even sent a card," and a colleague with whom he had worked for eighteen years "never called or wrote and to this day has never acknowledged my illness." And Victor Newton observed that "a few long-time friends stopped calling. . . . Some, I think, were simply afraid of cancer."[16]

After I had been diagnosed with prostate cancer, I looked over my holiday card register and my Rolodex and made lists. Family members and several close friends I called personally. Others I informed by a collective email, providing information about the biopsy results and my tentative plans for treatment. Most of the responses were enormously warm and supportive but, like others, I experienced a few people who appeared unable to deal with the subject in any form. You try to not take such reactions personally by reasoning that it is *their* problem.

COWORKERS AND BUSINESS COLLEAGUES

For many people, especially those living alone, their primary support network may be coworkers with whom they spend five days a week. They and business colleagues must be informed of your prostate cancer, and they can be very helpful. In your search for an appropriate doctor or hospital, for example, a coworker or business colleague may have a sister-in-law who works in a hospital or an uncle who had prostate cancer. Such individuals can markedly enlarge your information-gathering capacity. But they can't help with your cancer if they don't know you have it.

Handling news of your prostate cancer in the workplace is somewhat different from handling it among your friends. If you are a supervisor, the reaction of subordinates may vary from feeling threatened by the loss of their protector to being secretly pleased that they will be rid of you, at least for a while. As an employee, your medical leave is likely to put more work and responsibility onto others. For a man still in the prime of his career, a diagnosis of prostate cancer may make him a poor risk for further advancement. In general, this is not a major problem, for most people are aware that prostate cancers grow very slowly. One study showed that one year following treatment for prostate cancer, the employment rate for affected men did not differ from those not affected.[17] The Americans with Disabilities Act, passed in 1990, prohibits discrimination against employees for medical reasons, but the act is difficult to enforce.

After I had decided on a course of treatment and had a date for surgery, I personally told those with whom I was working most closely and then sent an email to the rest. It read as follows:

> To: All Concerned
> This is to let you know that I will be on medical leave for three weeks or so starting June 1. I will be having surgery for cancer of the prostate, which is not my first choice of how to spend time but better than other possible problems that come with age, such as Alzheimer's. It appears to be in a relatively early stage, so the long-term outlook is good.

I concluded with some humor, saying that I expected to receive get-well cards from two organizations that everyone was aware were the last organizations that would ever send cards to me. A general announcement of this sort seemed an effective way to avoid the whispering and rumors that routinely circulate in an office when some people know and others do not. It put everything on the table at once, and I found that within two or three days my working relationship with my coworkers had returned to normal.

Some coworkers and professional colleagues, of course, will be uncomfortable with any discussion of cancer. The differences may be cultural, since in some cultures and subcultures talking about cancer is still not polite. I discovered this myself when, three months after having surgery, I was at a professional meeting in Europe. Two of my European colleagues, whom I have known for many years, casually asked how I was, and I told them that I had recently been treated for prostate cancer. Their expressions and embarrassed reactions were similar to what I might have expected if I'd said I'd recently turned into a werewolf.

When confronted with professional colleagues and casual acquaintances I had not seen for a while, the issue of disclosure continued to be a dilemma. In response to the question "How are you doing?" I had to calculate how well I knew the person, whether they were likely to have heard about my cancer from others, and whether they even wanted to know. I found that there was no easy solution but that it became less of a problem over time.

SUPPORT GROUPS

For many men, prostate cancer support groups become their main support system. Properly run, such groups can be extremely helpful in providing information, friendship, and a place to discuss problems and side effects of treatment with others who have been there. Many men with prostate cancer derive satisfaction from helping others who are so affected.

These groups meet monthly or more often in a meeting room made available to them by a local hospital, community center, church, or synagogue. Some are led by professionals, usually a nurse or social worker, while others are led by the members themselves. Some groups are restricted to men only, whereas others include wives and partners. Groups may specialize in one area, such as men who have been recently diagnosed, men with recurrent cancer, or men with problems of incontinence or impotence.

There are two principal networks of prostate cancer support groups in the United States. Us Too, a network of over three hundred groups, is coordinated by Us Too International in Downer's Grove, Illinois. Local support groups can be identified on the Us Too website, www.ustoo.org, or by calling the Illinois office at 1-800-808-7866.

The other network of support groups is Man to Man, coordinated by the American Cancer Society. It was started in 1989 by a man who had grown tired of going to general cancer support groups in which most of the members were women. "I didn't want to hear

---

Support Groups

I think it's very valuable to belong to a support group. The more you talk about a problem you have, the easier it is to live with it. And you learn from other people. And if you talk about a subject, you're going to be more at ease, you're going to find out what's best to do and what's not.

—Charles Neider, *Adam's Burden*

---

about their cervix and they didn't want to hear about my prostate" was his impetus to begin the all-male groups. Local affiliates can be identified on the American Cancer Society website, www.cancer.org, or by calling the society's chapter in your area.

Many communities offer the two support groups, and men seeking help may wish to try both to see which better meets their needs. Support groups in Canada can be identified on the website of the Canadian Prostate Cancer Network, www.cpcn.org.

In summary, a support system is essential to assist you through prostate cancer. However, you are the key to developing that support, and it is primarily your responsibility to put it together. Family, friends, coworkers, and support group members can all be extremely helpful if you let them. The various members of your support system, in fact, are the initial elements in your healing process. Richard Handy described it nicely when he likened healing to the weaving of a tapestry:

> When a weaver first threads his loom, those individual bits of colors dotted at different locations seem to make no sense. But in time, with the addition of more strands and different loom settings, inchoate figures begin to emerge and grow into definite shapes. Only when the tapestry of my healing had been completed and I had stepped back several years later to see it completely, did the intricate architecture of its patterns, their interwoven themes and feelings, become clearer and better understood.[18]

10

Major Complications and Their Treatment

Incontinence and impotence are the two most-feared complications of prostate cancer treatment. They are the Scylla and
Charybdis of prostate voyagers, and rare is the man who successfully
sails by both without being affected by one or the other. Even men
who elect watchful waiting as their option may experience them as
their cancer increases in size. Although incontinence and impotence
have been briefly discussed in preceding chapters, their importance
for men with prostate cancer merits a chapter of their own.

It is vital, however, to place incontinence and impotence in
proper perspective. For men whose cancer has grown beyond the
prostate or spread to other organs, incontinence and impotence do
not loom so large. As Anatole Broyard noted: "In my own case, after a
brush with death, I feel that just to be alive is a permanent orgasm."[1]

Arguments abound about which is worse, incontinence or impotence. Walsh and Worthington, in their book *Dr. Patrick Walsh's
Guide to Surviving Prostate Cancer,* argue that "recovery of urine control is far more important and . . . casts a far greater shadow on your
life. If something's wrong with your ability to urinate, you'll be reminded of it several times a day—or worse, several times an hour—
not just a few times a week or month." On the other hand, many
men share the opinion of Charles Williams, who wrote that "not

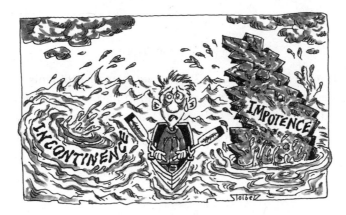

even the threat of death chilled me to the bone as much as the prospect of never being able to make love again." Many urologists agree that "once the dust settles on issues of cancer control and incontinence, erectile dysfunction is the lingering quality of life compromise for many men."[2] For any specific man, the choice of which is worse is usually easy to make: it is whichever affects him more.

URINARY INCONTINENCE: THE PROBLEM

Incontinence is a problem because the male urethra, which carries urine from the bladder to outside the body, runs directly through the prostate. Thus, when the prostate is being destroyed by surgery, radiation, or cryotherapy, the urethra is inevitably affected.

As detailed in Appendix A, urine flow in males is controlled by two sphincters—an internal one immediately above the prostate, where the urethra exits the bladder, and an external one just below the prostate. During surgery for prostate cancer, the internal sphincter is destroyed, because it is anatomically contiguous to the prostate; to preserve the internal sphincter risks leaving behind some cancer cells. That effectively leaves one working sphincter to do a job previously done by two. The average daily urine flow is approximately one-half gallon, so the task is demanding. Further, radiation and cryotherapy treatment may damage either or both sphincters.

The magnitude of urinary incontinence as a problem in any particular man depends on several factors. Most important is the function and strength of the external sphincter, the development of

---

An Incontinent House

One man noted that, while he was having problems with urinary incontinence, the plumbing in his house also developed problems. "The dishwasher leaked and stained the ceiling of the room below, the kitchen drain started dripping, a toilet seal had to be replaced, and the sink in the master bath joined the dripping chorus." He concluded, "My house is incontinent!"

—Aubrey Pilgrim,
A Revolutionary Approach to Prostate Cancer

---

which varies in different men. Like all muscles, it weakens with age. Urologists with lesser skills may inadvertently damage the external sphincter; the incontinence in such cases is caused by incompetence.

The two principal types of urinary incontinence are stress incontinence and urge incontinence. Stress incontinence occurs when pressure inside the abdomen increases, as during coughing, sneezing, blowing the nose, laughing, singing, passing gas, or exercising. The increased abdominal pressure causes the bladder to contract and thereby exert more pressure on the external sphincter, which, if it is weak, lets urine pass through. A full lower bowel will also cause this type of incontinence, since the bowel presses on the bladder.

Urge incontinence occurs when the man cannot hold his urine long enough to get to the bathroom. This may result from irritation or spasms of the bladder. It occurs frequently in men with benign prostatic hypertrophy and following radiation treatment for prostate cancer. Although most books discuss stress incontinence and urge incontinence as if they were distinctly separate entities, in real life many men have combinations of both types.

Assessing the severity of urinary incontinence is difficult because men vary widely in their reaction to it. Intermittent dribbling, necessitating the wearing of a thin pad, may be of no consequence for one man but a constant calamity for another. For this reason, Mark Litwin

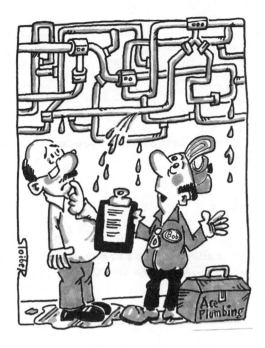

"This looks too complicated for me—I suggest
you call a urologist."

and his colleagues at UCLA Medical Center developed a brief questionnaire that covers both the magnitude of the problem and the
extent to which it bothers the man (see Table 6). The questionnaire is
now widely used because the correlation between the *magnitude* of
the problem and how much it *bothers* men turns out to be quite low;
that is, men with a small problem may be very bothered by it, and
men with a big problem may not be.

URINARY INCONTINENCE: THE SOLUTIONS

The good news about urinary incontinence caused by treatment for
prostate cancer is that in most cases the problem improves over time.
This is especially true of incontinence due to surgery, which initially may be a serious difficulty. Most studies suggest that incontinence continues to be a long-term major problem for approximately
5 to 10 percent of men treated for prostate cancer but can be improved with help.

Table 6. UCLA Prostate Cancer Index for Urinary Function

---

1. Over the LAST 4 WEEKS, how often have you leaked urine?

Every day 1   (Circle one number.)
About once a week 2
Less than once a week 3
Not at all 4

2. Which of the following best describes your urinary control *during the LAST 4 WEEKS?*

No control whatsoever 1   (Circle one number.)
Frequent dribbling 2
Occasional dribbling 3
Total control 4

3. How many pads or adult diapers per day did you usually use to control leakage *during the LAST 4 WEEKS?*

3 or more pads per day 1   (Circle one number.)
1–2 pads per day 2
No pads 3

4. How big a problem, if any, has each of the following been for you?

(Circle one number on each line.)	No problem	Very small problem	Small problem	Moderate problem	Big problem
a. Dripping urine or wetting your pants?	0	1	2	3	4
b. Urine leakage interfering with your sexual activity?	0	1	2	3	4

5. Overall, how big a problem has your urinary function been for you *during the LAST 4 WEEKS?*

No problem 1   (Circle one number.)
Very small problem 2
Small problem 3
Moderate problem 4
Big problem 5

SOURCE: Website of the UCLA Department of Urology (www.uclaurology.com); used with permission.

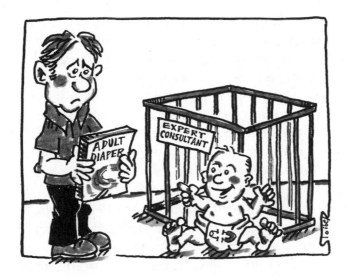

"That brand has excellent absorbency!"

The first step is to control the leakage with absorbent pads of some kind. A wide variety are available at pharmacies and medical supply stores. They range from what are essentially adult diapers to thin pads that can be tucked into one's underpants. The adult diapers are variously labeled as absorbent "underwear," "undergarments," or "fitted briefs" and are sold under brand names such as Attends, Depends, Poise, and Serenity. The next level down is underpants with an absorbent pouch in front, for instance, Sir Dignity briefs. As men develop increasing continence, they graduate to absorbent pads similar to those used by women during their menstrual periods. The pads come in a variety of sizes, shapes, and levels of absorbency, from extra plus, extra, and regular to light and ultra thin. Many have attachments and can be fitted easily into jockey-style underpants.

The next step in improving continence is to ask your urologist to rule out a urinary tract infection that could be making the problem worse. This can be done readily by checking the urine. In cases of severe and persistent incontinence, the urologist may want to carry out additional tests, such as putting a dye in the bladder and then viewing the bladder by X-ray (a cystogram) or by placing a thin tube up the penis to view the bladder (a cystoscopy).

Minimizing caffeine intake is a valuable step in controlling incontinence. Caffeine increases the frequency and urgency of having to urinate; thus, eliminating coffee, tea, and caffeine-containing soft drinks may improve matters. Medications being taken for other medical conditions may also worsen incontinence. Those known to do so include alpha-adrenergic blockers used to treat hypertension, including doxazosin (Cardura), prozasin (Minipress), and terazosin (Hytrin). Individuals taking these medications should ask their physicians to switch them to another type of antihypertensive medication.

Most urologists encourage patients undergoing prostate cancer treatment to do Kegel exercises to increase continence. These exercises were developed by Arnold Kegel in the 1940s for use by women who wanted to strengthen the muscles in the pelvis after childbirth. The difficulty is locating the correct muscles to be exercised. One set is used to stop urine flow; halting the flow in midstream and holding it for several seconds is the recommended way to identify these muscles. The other set is used to tighten the buttocks. One author suggests imagining that "you're trying to hold a quarter between your cheeks," while another, perhaps to greater effect, suggests the following:

> Imagine that you are standing on top of a hill, naked, with a $1,000 bill tucked between the cheeks of your buttocks. You are not able to use your hands, but you need to hold onto the bill during high gusty winds. That squeezing of your buttocks, pulling up internally and tightening down with your pelvic muscles, is a Kegel exercise.[3]

The true efficacy of Kegel exercises for men apparently has never been formally tested, so recommendations vary widely. Some urologists advise doing them "at least every hour for five minutes," while others suggest much less often. Some urologists say they should only be done standing up, while others urge doing them in any position, "while watching TV, driving a car, sitting in church, or anywhere at any time." Intriguingly, some claim that "Kegel exercises are also great for improving virility and achieving greater ejaculation and arousal control." In 2004 the National Institutes of Health funded a research project that is studying the best way to teach men to do Kegel exercises.[4]

Sometimes urinary continence can be modestly improved with medication. Decongestants, such as those used for colds, have been recommended; an example is pseudoephedrine (Sudafed). Imipramine (Tofranil), a commonly used antidepressant, may help the muscle tone of the sphincter. Oral anticholinergic drugs are widely used to improve continence in elderly persons and are worth trying; the most frequently prescribed are tolterodine (Detrol) and oxybutynin (Ditropan, Oxytrol). Dry mouth, blurred vision, constipation, and sleepiness are common side effects of anticholinergics. Men should always check with their urologist before starting on any of these drugs and ascertain that the new medication does not interact with those being taken for other conditions.

Despite all of the above suggestions, urinary incontinence will continue to be a problem for 5 to 10 percent of men following prostate cancer treatment. Injections of collagen through the urethra may strengthen the sphincter for approximately half of the men who try it, but it is expensive and the effects are usually not lasting. Out of desperation, some men use a foam rubber penile clamp, which can be released when the man wishes to urinate, or a condom catheter (widely known as a Texas catheter), which is worn on the penis and collects the urine, but both solutions bring their own complications and are not recommended by most urologists.

The definitive solution for severe, prolonged urinary incontinence is an artificial sphincter. It can be surgically implanted around the urethra and operated by a small bulb placed in the scrotum. When the man wishes to urinate, he squeezes the bulb, which opens the urethra; after a minute or two the sphincter automatically closes again. Despite its high cost and possible complications, such as infection and the need for replacement, the artificial sphincter has given a normal life back to many men previously plagued by incontinence.

My own experience with incontinence was fortunately brief. I found it strange and embarrassing to buy what is essentially an adult diaper but was impressed by how much pharmacy shelf space was allotted to these items; I was reassured that I had plenty of company! Luckily, my external sphincter took charge almost immediately after removal of the catheter, and I was able to discard the adult diaper and heavy pads within a day. By the end of three weeks I did not require any pad, and thereafter have had only occasional minor dribbling when I increase my abdominal pressure. The dribbling is less than what I experienced in the years immediately prior to surgery. Al-

The Artificial Sphincter:
A Paean to No Longer Being Peed On

It isn't until after a shower the next morning that I begin to feel like a whole person again. Save for the quirky little maneuver I have to go through to urinate, it is a heady feeling to feel like the same man I was before. No more a prisoner locked in solitary, I can walk in the sunlight, free of the Velcro shackles.

I'm neither a nudist, nor have I flasher tendencies, but it is a thrill to be able to walk around without anything on. Not to be able to perform the simple, most natural act of walking naked from a shower to a bedroom a few feet away can only be described as living in a cell without walls; it is days before I can allow myself to appreciate their disappearance. . . .

I sleep deeply, dream-free and, not since the night before the first operation, in the raw. The nightmare is over. I think I can hear the fat lady singing.

—Bert Gottlieb, describing what it's like to
have an artificial sphincter, in *The Men's Club*

though radical prostatectomy is much more likely to *cause* urinary incontinence than to *improve* it, studies have shown that for some men the surgery does, in fact, improve urinary symptoms.[5]

IMPOTENCE: THE PROBLEM

Impotence, or erectile dysfunction (ED), as it has become known, is the gorilla in the prostate cancer closet. It lurks just out of sight but never out of mind. Choosing between various treatments for prostate cancer based on the likelihood of impotence is a little like choosing how you wish to die—the outcome of all the choices is remarkably similar.

Normal male sexual functioning is complex. A man must feel

some desire—libido—and this urge is instigated by a mix of testosterone and psychological factors. The penis must become erect, which is determined by the arteries, veins, and nerves that supply it. Orgasm is initiated in the brain and involves the ejaculation of sperm and seminal fluid through the contraction of muscles. And all of this must be orchestrated smoothly if it is to be successful.

The problem in cases of prostate cancer is that the arteries, veins, and nerves that control erections run alongside the prostate. To treat prostate cancer by any method means risking damage to one or more of these. The arteries are needed to carry blood to the penis. The nerves cause the smooth muscles in the penis to relax so that it can fill with blood. This filling, in turn, shuts the veins, thereby trapping blood in the penis. An erection, therefore, is simply a penis engorged with blood, and erectile dysfunction occurs when blood does not fill the penis as it is supposed to. Even when a nerve-sparing procedure is used in the surgical removal of the prostate, arteries and veins may still be damaged, with resultant erectile dysfunction.

More misinformation probably exists about sexual function than about any other aspect of prostate cancer. One man was told that treatment would "have no physiological effect on my libido or sensation of orgasm. . . . I would still be able to achieve orgasm, and it would feel much the same as before." A widely read book reassures men that after a radical prostatectomy, they will have "normal sensation, normal sex drive, and can achieve a normal orgasm." And, even if they do have erectile dysfunction, it "can always be treated."[6]

The truth is quite different. Certain men have been shown to experience a decrease in libido following treatment for prostate cancer, although it is usually not marked. Some of the decrease may be due to a lessening of testosterone, although the mechanism for this decrease is not clear. Diminished libido may also be due to depression secondary to erectile dysfunction or other factors.

Ejaculation is abolished by prostate surgery, since the seminal vesicles, which supply most of the seminal fluid, and the vasa deferentia, which carry the sperm, are both severed. As one man noted, ejaculation was "visible proof of my manhood. . . . And now that integral part of my sexual expression was going to be taken away from me forever. . . . No semen, no ejaculation! It was as cut and dried as a beheading." As George Burns described it when, in his early 90s, he was asked about his sexual performance: "I come dust." One man who had prostate surgery looked on the humorous side of not ejaculating: "Now that I would no longer produce my ejaculate, I might even be able to fake an orgasm."[7] Ejaculation is also decreased by radiation treatments, although this effect takes place more slowly.

For most men the quality of orgasms is less intense after treatment for prostate cancer—hardly surprising, given the number of pelvic structures affected by the surgery. The same is true after radiation treatment. Michael Dorso, a physician who elected radiation treatment for his prostate cancer, wrote: "I really miss my prostate gland! . . . What I didn't realize is that it produces about 80% of the pleasure of an ejaculation. That feel-good pulsing in my groin during orgasm is gone!"[8]

The principal loss in sexual function after prostate cancer treatment is the ability to achieve an erection sufficient for intercourse. Charles Neider calls it having joined "the Limp Penis Club."[9] As noted in previous chapters, it now seems clear that the majority of men who undergo prostate cancer treatment of any kind will suffer some degree of erectile dysfunction.

Are there any predictors regarding which men are more likely to develop such dysfunction? The first key predictor is age. As men grow older, they progressively lose some of the nerves that supply the penis; in addition, the arteries, like arteries elsewhere in the body, may function less well. According to one estimate, "by age 60, a man only has about sixty percent of the nerves he was born with."[10]

The second major predictor of sexual function following treatment for prostate cancer is the man's sexual functioning prior to treatment. Studies have reported that approximately 20 percent of adult men are unable to achieve erections sufficient for vaginal intercourse, and an additional 30 percent have difficulty maintaining erections.[11] The reality, therefore, is that at least one third of men suffer some degree of erectile dysfunction at the time they are diagnosed with prostate cancer; such men are certainly not going to function better after treatment. The scenario reminds me of the man who asked his urologist whether he would be able to play the piano after having prostate surgery. "I don't see why not," said the urologist. "Why, that's wonderful," said the man. "I never could play before."

The third predictor of posttreatment erectile dysfunction is

Is It Possible to Accurately Assess Erectile Dysfunction after Prostate Cancer Treatment?

It is difficult to get credible figures on the incidence of erectile dysfunction following prostate cancer treatment, in part because many men do not answer such questions honestly. Assessments also vary depending on the definitions used. Does a man qualify as having an erection if his penis, which normally hangs at 7 o'clock, reaches 8:30 or 9 o'clock? Does it depend on how stiff it is? Or how long the erection lasts? Or whether he can only get an erection while standing up? Or only with the assistance of medication? Some have defined an erection as one sufficient to achieve vaginal penetration, but that depends in part on the partner's anatomy and cooperation. And what about frequency—if one achieves an erection once every six months, is that sufficient to say that erectile dysfunction does not exist?

Urologists who advocate for one or another form of treatment assess erectile dysfunction differently in attempts to make their numbers look good. Their data are often not reliable.

whether the man has other causes of dysfunction. Diabetes often contributes, and many medications cause a degree of erectile dysfunction, including some of those taken for hypertension and depression. It is often possible for a man to substitute another medication that has fewer such side effects.

The final predictor of erectile dysfunction following prostate cancer treatment is the type of treatment the man received. Surgical prostatectomy produces immediate erectile dysfunction in almost all cases but then a slow recovery of function, peaking at eighteen to twenty-four months. Recovery is most likely when both nerves were spared but, at least in one study, almost as satisfactory when only one nerve is spared.[12] Radiation produces little erectile dysfunction initially, but such dysfunction increases over the following months and even years. Cryotherapy and hormone therapy produce the most erectile dysfunction.

One other aspect of erectile dysfunction following prostate cancer treatment is rarely discussed: the possible loss of the man's sexual fantasy life. A study among forty-eight men who had been treated by surgery, beam, and seed radiation therapy reported the following:

> The men became nostalgic when they described how they once enjoyed thinking about sex, now a lost pastime. They disclosed that they no longer enjoyed sexual feelings in response to seeing an attractive woman. They also expressed a profound sense of loss associated with a loss of a fantasy life in which they were able to imagine themselves as potential sexual partners. They were sadly conscious of their diminished libidos.[13]

These men had previously enjoyed seeing attractive women in their everyday lives and fantasizing about them. The experience was "something that they had identified as part of their lives as men." Impotence, however, rendered these fantasies unrealistic. This study makes clear that a man's loss of potency following prostate cancer treatment leads to more than erectile dysfunction; it may lead to "fantasy dysfunction as well." For some men, this can be a serious loss.

IMPOTENCE: THE SOLUTIONS

The importance of having an active sex life varies widely among men, especially among men of different ages. For a man who is diagnosed with prostate cancer in his 40s and who has a younger wife, the threat of impotence may appear catastrophic. For a man in his 60s, with a wife of similar age, the threat of impotence following treatment for prostate cancer may be something he can live with, especially if he believes that the treatment has cured his cancer. This willingness to accept partial or full impotence in exchange for a successful cancer treatment may explain why, in one survey, "nearly half the men who experience erectile dysfunction after prostate cancer therapy choose not to seek treatment for their impotence."[14] It

Adjusting to Impotence

I could not predict just how the loss of . . . sexual potency might affect me. I was certain it would not enhance my self-image, but perhaps I would handle it reasonably well. Important as it was in my life, sexual activity did not involve large blocks of my time on a daily basis. Most of what gives meaning—family, friends, teaching, reading, writing, movies, bicycling, squash, skiing, good food—would still be there and there was little reason to think that my capacity for any of them, with the short-term exception of bicycling, would be diminished in any way.

—William Martin, *My Prostate and Me*

Patients can have excellent quality of life even though erections and urinary control may not be perfect. I'm sure that there are many patients who have artificial hips and knees who cannot run and dance like they once did but are pleased with the outcome.

—Patrick Walsh, letter, *Journal of Urology*, 2004

may also explain the wide disparity reported by researchers between men who are deeply distressed by posttreatment sexual dysfunction and men who are little bothered by the dysfunction.

A critical step in finding solutions to the impotence problem is open and frank discussion between the man and his partner. Michael Dorso advises that "the silent male model doesn't work here" and adds:

Men seem to have more trouble than women talking about their intimate feelings and erotic needs. You will have to overcome your chauvinistic leanings. It seems to be one of life's paradoxes, that sometimes a frank sexual discussion can be most difficult with the one sharing our bed! Bizarre, isn't it? You may have looked into her eyes as you shared thousands of orgasms, and yet find it difficult to look into her eyes and discuss your new sexual concerns.[15]

There are many ways to enhance whatever erectile function remains after prostate cancer treatment. Direct physical stimulation of the penis by the man or his partner is more effective than visual or fantasy stimulation. It can be assisted by lubricants such as K-Y jelly, Astroglide, or, least expensive of all, saliva. A standing position often helps erections, making it more difficult for blood to escape from the penis and return uphill to the heart. Another means of slowing the escape of blood is to place a rubber band or erection ring, available in sex shops, around the base of the penis prior to foreplay. Blood can then enter the penis through the central arteries but can less readily escape through the weaker-walled veins, which are constricted by the bands.

Even men who have complete erectile dysfunction can have a sex life after prostate cancer treatment. Since orgasms begin in the brain, not the penis, they are still possible, although they may be more difficult to achieve. As in all aspects of sexual function, practice makes perfect. People's physical needs and responses differ. As one author notes: "Just as all artists have to practice with different brushes and mixing colors and how to apply them to get the desired result, if we want to improve our lovemaking, we have to do the same."[16] It has been said that as we deal with the problem of a flexible penis, it is best not to be too rigid; in fact, flexibility often produces greater rigidity.

Articles, books, and website advice abound regarding how to improve sexual functioning following prostate cancer treatment. Among the best sources of information is *The Lovin' Ain't Over: The Couples Guide to Better Sex after Prostate Disease,* by Ralph and Barbara Alterowitz (see Appendix B). The premise of the book is that "you can have a loving and satisfying sexual relationship without having an erection." They suggest:

> Don't focus on the erection. Instead, focus on loving and deriving pleasure from it. When erections were easy, we tended to focus solely on them. In reality, most of us missed out on other means of deriving pleasure, which could have made loving much more pleasurable even then.

Masturbation: Sweet Irony!

Authorities agree that exercising the penis early and often following treatment for prostate cancer increases the chances for return of function. The penis needs an abundant blood supply to nourish the tissues, and the arteries to the penis are often damaged during treatment. Books advocate activities such as frequent "direct sexual stimulation" and "penile massage."

Many of us older men remember hearing in our youths that masturbation was "self-abuse" and would make us become blind. I recall the story of the boy who was caught masturbating by his mother and told to stop. "But mother, can't I continue just until I need glasses?" he replied.

But now, sweet irony! In our youth, we were told that masturbation would cause a deterioration of our body. In our old age, we are now told that *not* masturbating will cause a deterioration of our body.

Similarly, Michael Dorso notes that "making love does not have to equal sex; furthermore having sex does not have to equal intercourse." Women know this better than men do and, judging from comments posted on prostate cancer websites, it seems to be a difficult lesson for men to learn. Dorso's wife put it most succinctly: "Michael, I married you for who you are, not for your penis."[17]

For men who want to enhance their erections with artificial means, the five main options are oral medications, penile injections, vacuum pumps, nerve grafts, and surgically implantable penile prostheses. Of these, oral medications are by far the most popular and most widely used. It is, in fact, difficult to watch a sporting event on television without seeing advertisements for sildenafil (Viagra), vardenafil (Levitra), or tadalafil (Cialis). These medications are helpful for many men, but they do not live up to the promise of instant pharmaceutical nirvana that the ads suggest. In one study of their

Oral Medications to Enhance Erections

sildenafil (Viagra)
- 25 mg., 50 mg., and 100 mg. rectangular blue tablets
- peak action 30 minutes to 2 hours; may last up to 6 hours
- food affects action, so should not be taken less than one hour before or within two hours after eating

vardenafil (Levitra)
- 2.5 mg, 5 mg, 10 mg, and 20 mg round white tablets
- peak action 30 minutes to 2 hours; may last up to 12 hours
- okay to take with food except for high-fat meals, which delay onset of action

tadalafil (Cialis)
- 5 mg, 10 mg, and 20 mg oval sand-colored tablets
- peak action 30 minutes to 6 hours; may last up to 36 hours
- okay to take with food

Side effects: All three medications can have similar side effects: flushing, headache, dizziness, indigestion, and stuffy nose. Sildenafil also occasionally gives a blue tinge to vision. Rarely, the medications may produce a prolonged erection (priapism), which should be treated with ice packs and, if needed, a visit to the emergency room, or they may cause some loss of vision, which may be permanent.

DO NOT TAKE these medications if you are also taking *nitrate* medications for angina or chest pain. The combination can cause a severe fall in blood pressure and even death. (The nitrate drugs include isosorbide, Dilatrate, Isordil, Sorbitrate, Ismo, Imdur, nitroglycerin, Deponit, Minitran, Nitro-Bid, Nitrodisc, Nitro-Dur, Nitrostat, and Transderm-Nitro.)

You should start at a low dose and take the new drugs cautiously if you are also taking any of the following:
- medications to lower blood pressure, especially doxazosin (Cardura)

- medications for benign prostatic hypertrophy, such as tamsulosin (Flomax)
- medications for AIDS
- erythromycin, ketoconazole (Nizoral), itraconazole (Sporanox)
- antidepressants in the selective serotonin reuptake inhibitor category (SSRIs)

efficacy in men who had had a radical prostatectomy, they were said to be helpful two thirds of the time in men younger than age 55 but only one third of the time in men 60 or older.[18]

The oral medications, first introduced in 1997, work by blocking an enzyme (phosphodiesterase type 5) in the penis, thereby allowing the smooth muscles to relax and the penis to fill with blood. They do not produce an erection by themselves, but only when accompanied by erotic stimulation. The effective dose varies among men; some men, but not all, get a better response at a higher dose. These medications should *never be taken by men who are also taking nitrates for angina or chest pain;* the drug interaction can be fatal.

Another rare but important side effect is their propensity for causing blurred vision and/or partial blindness, usually in one eye, a condition officially called nonarteric ischemic optic neuropathy (NAION). At least forty cases have been reported, and the eye changes are usually permanent. Men who have hypertension, diabetes, hyperlipidemia, and/or a small optic cup (which can be assessed via an exam by an ophthalmologist or optician) are at higher risk for this side effect.[19]

No controlled studies have yet been done comparing the three medications. If a man does not respond to one of them, it is not clear what his chances are of responding to another one. All three medications are priced similarly, at approximately $10 per pill.

Some research has suggested that oral medications to enhance erections not only have an immediate benefit—a stronger erection—but may also have longer-term benefits by preventing fibrosis and atrophy of penile tissue. Biopsies of penile tissue were performed at six-month intervals in two groups of men: one group took sildenafil every other night for six months and the other did not.[20] If additional, longer-term benefits are definitely proven, these medications will be routinely prescribed to preserve penile function in men undergoing treatment for cancer of the prostate.

Another form of the same type of medication can be placed directly into the urethra as a suppository. Called MUSE (Medicated Urethral System for Erection), it has been used less since the oral medications became widely available.

Men for whom oral medications are not effective may choose to try injections directly into the penis. The medications dilate the blood vessels, allowing the penis to fill with blood, and may produce a serviceable erection lasting for about an hour. Self-injection is not for all men, however, and, as noted by one author, "obviously is not ideal for men who can't see well [and] men with poor hand-eye coordination."[21] Penile self-injections are well described by Robert Hitchcock in *Love, Sex, and PSA* and by Michael Korda in *Man to Man* (see Appendix B).

The other three options for erection enhancement are vacuum pumps, nerve grafts, and penile prosthetic implants. The pump is placed over the penis prior to intercourse and, by creating a vacuum, draws blood into it. Some men find it quite satisfactory, while others do not; for example, Charles Neider complained that "the penis doesn't seem to be sensitive" and "it's erect, but not stiff."[22] Nerve grafts are still experimental and are usually done at the time of surgery on men in whom neither nerve can be saved. Penile prosthetic implants must be inserted by a surgeon and come in a variety of styles. Chuck Wheeler in *Affirming the Darkness* describes having such an implant. Vacuum pumps and implants are both explained in detail in Sheldon Marks's *Prostate and Cancer* and Paul Lange and Christine Adamec's *Prostate Cancer for Dummies* (see Appendix B).

My own experience with erectile dysfunction has been reasonably satisfactory. Like most men, I had almost complete erectile dysfunction immediately following surgery. After a few weeks, I was able to achieve orgasm, but, as noted by others, it was less intense than before. The initial orgasms were accompanied by minor pelvic pain and some loss of urine; both have been described by other men, and both resolved spontaneously.

I found vardenafil (Levitra) to be the most helpful of the three available oral medications. Other aids were a standing position, which forces the blood in the penis to run uphill to the heart; a rubber band at the base of the penis to partially constrict the veins and thereby slow the outflow of blood; and sexual activity in the morning hours, when it is known that testosterone levels, and thus libido, are highest.

I noted a slow improvement in erectile function between three and six months postsurgery, at which time I successfully had vaginal intercourse. I had mentally prepared myself to possibly never have this experience again, so it was a memorable event. Between six and twelve months, erectile progress was more rapid. According to one study, the maximal erection recovery following prostate cancer surgery does not occur until after an average of eighteen months, but it can continue for two years or longer.[23]

Despite all of the available aids for recovering erectile function, the single most important factor, in my experience, is having a loving and understanding wife or partner. In this, I feel truly fortunate and would wish the same for every man who must confront recovery from prostate cancer.

11

What Happens if the Cancer
Spreads or Comes Back?

Living with prostate cancer, said one man, is "like being trapped inside a cage with a baby lion." In the beginning, the lion is small and nonthreatening, but you know that the lion will grow and may eventually devour you. This man's cancer did spread and in the end did "devour" him.[1]

Prior to the PSA era, by the time of diagnosis the prostate cancer would have already spread beyond the prostate in the majority of cases. By the 1990s, this number had been reduced to one third, and by now it is presumably significantly lower than that.

Prostate cancers that have spread at the time of diagnosis present many of the same treatment problems as cancers that recur after the initial treatment. In some cases, the recurrence is expected because of a Gleason score of 8 to 10, a PSA over 20, or other indicators of a large and serious cancer. In other cases, the recurrence of the cancer is unexpected, as when a man has a low Gleason score, a low PSA, and a small tumor. Some of these men are told by their urologists that they are "cured" following their initial surgical or radiation treatments, and recurrence of the cancer, when it occurs, can be a cruel shock.

It is helpful to keep in mind the magnitude of the recurrence problem. There are approximately 1.6 million men in the United States who have been diagnosed with and, in most cases, treated

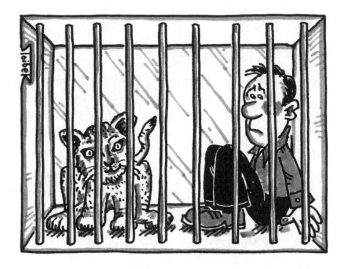

for prostate cancer. They constitute 17 percent of Americans who are living with cancer. The majority of these men have regular PSA checks at least annually for ten to fifteen years. Each time they are tested, they wait nervously for the results—will this be the time their PSA is elevated, indicating the recurrence of cancer? Since the recurrence of prostate cancer is often without symptoms, there is a Kafkaesque quality to the repeat PSA tests, a mysterious internal process over which a man has no control.

WILL IT KILL ME, AND IF SO, WHEN?

The recurrence and spread of prostate cancer usually follow certain pathways. If the cancer was removed surgically, microscopic bits of cancer may have been left behind where the prostate lay (called the bed of the prostate). If the cancer was treated with radiation, it may recur in portions of the prostate that did not receive enough radiation to kill all the cancer cells. At any point, the cancer may spread beyond the prostate to the seminal vesicles, adjacent lymph nodes, or bladder; this is called local spread. It may also spread more distantly, called metastasis. Bones, especially the spine, are favorite sites for prostate cancer metastases, but late in its course the cancer may also metastasize to the kidneys or virtually anywhere in the body.

The predictors of prostate cancer spread include the same factors

A Clerk in a Great Court

I try not to think about the number but I can't help doing it. PSA is like a clerk in a great court sitting in judgment on me, on my health or illness, my life or death. What terrible or wonderful message will this clerk deliver? Will I be condemned? Or rescued? And will the tumor be smaller? If so, how small? Will my side effects have been experienced in vain? Did I make a serious mistake in not selecting a prostatectomy? Or watchful waiting? Wait, wait, wait and see.

—Charles Neider, *Adam's Burden*

that predict a serious cancer. Men who have a PSA greater than 20, a Gleason score of 8 to 10, or a large tumor that occupies both lobes of the prostate are at high risk for recurrence. Thus, a man with a PSA between 4 and 10 has an 11 percent chance of cancer recurrence at five years, whereas a man with a PSA over 20 has a 40 percent chance; in addition, the man with the higher PSA will have his cancer recur sooner. Similarly, a man with a Gleason score of 6 or less has a 3 percent chance of recurrence at five years, whereas a man with a Gleason score of 8 to 10 has a 38 percent chance. A man whose cancer occupies more than 20 percent of the prostate has three times the risk of recurrence as a man whose cancer occupies less than 10 percent of the gland.[2]

Several efforts have been made to put various factors together into a single schema to predict prostate cancer spread following surgery or radiation treatment. These schema are referred to as nomograms, which are merely graphic representations of risk based on the past experience of similar men. The simplest nomogram for men following surgery consists of the following:[3]

- Take your numerical Gleason score.
- Add 1 if your PSA was 4 to 10.
- Add 2 if your PSA was 10.1 to 20.

- Add 3 if your PSA was over 20.
- Add 2 if your seminal vesicles were positive for cancer at surgery.
- Add 2 if the cancer had positive margins at surgery.
- Subtract 4 if you had add-on (adjuvant) hormone treatment.
- Subtract 2 if you had add-on (adjuvant) radiation treatment.

Add the numbers. Your chances that your cancer will recur, as measured by rising PSA five years following surgery, are shown in Table 7.

Additional nomograms, developed by Michael Kattan and his colleagues at Memorial Sloan-Kettering Cancer Center in New York, are widely used by physicians and are commonly referred to as Kattan tables.[4] The nomograms utilize information such as size of the cancer and evidence of invasion at surgery, or radiation dose and length of radiation therapy. A major shortcoming of all systems is that they are based on the experience of men treated in past years, whereas treatments are continuing to improve and past experience may not necessarily be applicable.

There are three main stages in the recurrence and spread of prostate cancer:

1. *Recurrence as measured by PSA*: As noted in Chapters 3 and 4, a rise in the PSA after surgical or radiation treatment indicates recurrence of cancer. In the medical literature, this increase is commonly referred to as a biochemical failure. If the PSA is going to rise in a postsurgical patient, it will do so within the first five years in 72 percent of cases; between five and ten years in 23 percent of cases; and between ten and fifteen years in 5 percent of cases. It is rare to have a recurrence of cancer beyond fifteen years. Or we might say that the average time from surgery to a rising PSA is three and a half years.[5]

Once the cancer has recurred, as indicated by a rise in the PSA, its progression is highly variable. If no treatment is given, the PSA will continue to rise relatively rapidly in approximately half of all men, slowly in a third of men, and very slowly in the remainder. In 7 percent of cases, the PSA will not reach a level of 10 in less than twenty years.[6] Thus, some men will have a continuously rising PSA and progression of their cancer, while others will have almost no progression for many years despite receiving no treatment.

Table 7. Nomogram for Predicting Recurrence of Cancer
Five Years Following Surgery

Total points	Percent recurrence
5 or less	6%
6	10
7	18
8	23
9	33
10	40
11	48
12	60
13 or more	68

2. *Progression from PSA rise to metastasis*: The single best predictor of the continuing progression of recurrent prostate cancer is the PSA doubling time. As the name implies, this is the time it takes for the PSA level to go, for example, from 1.1 to 2.2 or 4.2 to 8.4. The shorter the doubling time, the worse the prognosis for men treated by either surgery or radiation. If the PSA doubles in less than six months, it is likely that the cancer has already metastasized to bones or other organs; if it doubles in more than twelve months, the cancer is probably still localized near the prostate bed.

Charles Pound and his colleagues at Johns Hopkins University developed predictions of how long it takes recurrent prostate cancer to metastasize once the PSA has risen, based on the PSA doubling time, Gleason score, and whether the initial PSA rise occurred sooner than two years after surgery (see Table 8).[7]

Having a shorter PSA doubling time doubles the chances that a man will have metastases by seven years after the PSA rise, other things being equal. Note that these predictions are a best-case scenario, since they represent the outcome for 304 men who were an average age of 58 when operated on for prostate cancer. There is evidence that younger men with prostate cancer have a better prognosis, so older men are likely to have a higher rate of metastasis than these numbers predict. Among the men followed at Johns Hopkins, the median time from PSA rise to metastasis was eight years, but varied from two to twelve years.

3. *Progression from metastasis to death*: The interval between the

Table 8. Percentage of Prostate Cancers That Will Have Spread to Bones or Other Organs, as Predicted by PSA Doubling Time, Gleason Score, and How Quickly the PSA Rose Following Surgery

PSA doubling time:	Gleason scores 5–7; PSA rise more than two years after surgery		
	at 3 years	at 5 years	at 7 years
more than 10 months	5%	14%	18%
less than 10 months	18%	31%	40%

PSA doubling time:	Gleason scores 5–7; PSA rise less than two years after surgery		
	at 3 years	at 5 years	at 7 years
more than 10 months	21%	24%	41%
less than 10 months	19%	65%	85%

	Gleason scores 8–10; PSA rise more than two years after surgery		
	at 3 years	at 5 years	at 7 years
	23%	40%	53%

	Gleason scores 8–10; PSA rise less than two years after surgery		
	at 3 years	at 5 years	at 7 years
	47%	69%	79%

NOTE: The numbers are based on 304 men who had a rise in their PSA following radical prostatectomy at Johns Hopkins Hospital between 1982 and 1997. The average age of the men at surgery was 58. Younger men generally have a more benign course than older men; thus, these predictions may be overly optimistic for older men.
SOURCE: C. R. Pound, A. W. Partin, M. A. Eisenberger, et al., Natural history of progression after PSA elevation following radical prostatectomy, *Journal of the American Medical Association* 281 (1999): 1591–97.

development of prostate cancer metastases and death averages three to five years in various studies. In the Johns Hopkins study cited above, the median time was five years, but as noted, it was a study of younger men. The Pound group found that the shorter the interval between surgery and the development of metastases, the shorter the time to death was likely to be. For example, among men who developed metastases within three years of surgery, 87 percent had died by five years after their surgery.[8]

> ### Stages of Disease
>
> The distinction between stages of disease is an arbitrary one. There is no single moment when Victor's cancer ceased to be something he lived with and became, instead, something that was killing him. It was killing him from the beginning and he lived with it until the end. Still, there is some reason to divide the experience into periods. There was a time when Victor lived a more or less normal life despite the disease, and it was followed by a period that was not like normal life at all, when we understood that his life itself was nearing its end. There was no defining moment that separated one period from the other, but they were nonetheless different.
>
> —Audrey Newton, *Living with Prostate Cancer*

In summary, the sooner the PSA rises following treatment for prostate cancer, the worse the prognosis. Thereafter, the faster the PSA doubling time, the sooner the man is likely to develop metastases. And the sooner he develops metastases, the sooner he is likely to die. The duration from initial treatment to rise in PSA averages three to four years but may be as long as fifteen years. The duration from PSA rise to metastasis averages six to eight years, and from metastasis to death three to five years. Thus, for men whose cancer appears not to have spread at the time of initial diagnosis, the average time between initial treatment and death will be approximately fifteen years for those who are destined to die from their cancer. This prediction is not valid for men whose cancer has already spread at the time of initial diagnosis.

Always keep in mind, however, that predictions are merely predictions. As in all recurrent cancers, one subgroup progresses very rapidly, one subgroup progresses hardly at all, and the vast majority of men fall between these two extremes. There are always those who defy predictions. Consider the 45-year-old man who in 1976 was diagnosed with prostate cancer that had already metastasized to his

bones and distant lymph nodes. He was treated with hormone therapy and twenty-seven years later was still doing fine.[9] All of us who
have prostate cancer hope that we too will do better than the average
predictions.

TREATMENT OPTIONS FOR RECURRENT CANCER

There are two goals in treating prostate cancer that has spread: (1) improve the quantity of the man's life, and (2) improve the quality of
the man's life. The dilemmas in treatment arise when attempts to
improve quantity make the quality worse, not better. Honest assessments of treatment options are crucial to resolving these dilemmas.

The mainstay for treating recurrent prostate cancer is hormone
therapy, as described in Chapter 5. Prostate cancers use testosterone
to grow, so blocking testosterone slows the growth. Prostate cancers
contain cells that are sensitive to testosterone and other cells that are
not sensitive. Over time the testosterone-insensitive cells become
predominant and hormone therapy becomes ineffective. The cancer
is then called androgen independent. The average duration of effectiveness for hormone therapy for a prostate cancer that has already
metastasized is approximately two years,[10] but during that time men
often have comfortable remissions.

One of the two major controversies in providing hormone therapy to men with recurrent prostate cancer concerns when to start the
treatment: as soon as the PSA rises, or not until the cancer metasta-
sizes or otherwise causes symptoms of growth. Proponents of immediate treatment point to two studies reporting that immediate hormone therapy produced better outcomes. In one study, men treated
with immediate hormone therapy, compared to those for whom
hormone therapy was delayed, developed metastases more slowly,
had half the number of serious complications (pathological fractures, spinal cord compression, obstructions of the ureter), and survived longer. In the other study, at seven years after treatment only
6 percent (3 of 47) of the men who had received immediate hormone
therapy had died from prostate cancer compared to 31 percent (16 of
51) of the men who had received delayed therapy.[11]

Proponents of delayed hormone therapy point to an older study
that had results exactly opposite to the two studies cited above. They

also argue that giving hormones to men before there is evidence of cancer spread means subjecting them unnecessarily to the multiple side effects of hormones. Patrick Walsh, a staunch opponent of immediate hormone therapy, says that it "will actually take life out of the years a man has to live, without adding any years to that life." Walsh also notes that the pharmaceutical industry has strongly influenced urologists to start hormone therapy early because the industry "makes at least a billion dollars a year on hormonal agents for the treatment of prostate cancer."[12] Several studies are under way that perhaps will resolve the immediate versus delayed treatment debate.

The other active hormone therapy controversy is whether to give hormones continuously or intermittently (in other words, treat the man for a few months until his PSA falls and then stop treatment for several months until the PSA rises again). The two arguments for intermittent therapy are that it gives the man a better quality of life by giving him a "vacation" from the hormone therapy side effects, and that intermittent therapy delays the process of the cancer's becoming androgen independent.

Some but not all studies support these arguments. A European study reported that only 7 percent of men on intermittent hormone therapy had had progression of their cancer at the end of three years compared to 39 percent of the men on continuous hormone therapy. A U.S. study found no difference in progression rates between the two groups. There does appear to be consensus that the quality of life is better for men on intermittent therapy, since they have periods free from the side effects of the therapy;[13] therefore, intermittent therapy is being increasingly used. Two large studies comparing continuous and intermittent hormone therapy are in progress.

Beam radiation is the second most commonly used treatment for men who have recurrent prostate cancer. It can be utilized in one of three ways. First, as what is commonly referred to as adjuvant therapy, beam radiation can be used immediately following surgery to radiate the prostate bed in men at high risk for cancer recurrence—say, with a Gleason score of 8 to 10. At least ten studies have suggested that this therapy may reduce, or at least delay, the chances of recurrence of cancer.[14] Radiating the prostate bed after surgery, however, carries with it an inevitable increase in incontinence,

Intermittent Hormone Therapy

I was first diagnosed with prostate cancer at the tender age of 36. Subsequently, . . . I went through the conventional treatments of radical prostatectomy and . . . radiation therapy to the prostate bed. . . . Five years later in 1989 I was faced with a new problem: It became apparent that my PSA . . . was rising significantly. . . . The conventional wisdom at the time was for me to undergo immediate castration—a more than terrifying prospect especially for a psychiatrist like myself with some background in studying Freud. . . . [A urologist suggested intermittent hormone therapy.] Instead of my facing a permanent blockade of testosterone, this protocol lasts for only nine months at a time, followed by two years of normal testosterone levels. His recommendation has proved to be objectively correct. Friends and colleagues who underwent permanent castration when facing a similar bind at the same time have all since died.

—Paul Steinberg, "Safety in Numbers,"
Washington Post, August 24, 2004

impotence, rectal bleeding, and other side effects. And since it is not known which cancers are going to recur, many men are unnecessarily irradiated.

The second use of beam radiation for cancer recurrence is called salvage radiation therapy. It is utilized once the PSA rises, indicating that recurrence has taken place. The radiation is directed at the prostate bed, where it is assumed some prostate tissue is growing. This approach has become increasingly popular as the first choice for treatment when cancer recurs after surgery, with many men saving hormone therapy for later use if needed. Although no studies have yet demonstrated that salvage beam radiation prevents the development of metastases or lengthens life, several studies have reported promising results: one large study found that 45 percent of the men

---

Is God Besotted with Irony?

I do get profoundly sad thinking of what has been and is no longer: people, places, things. And in my art I've tried again and again to find ways to hold on to the precious in the present, to memorialize what is essential to me as an observer of my time, to make history come alive so that souls long dead will still have meaning. Indeed, is it not wonderfully ironic that I worked for twenty-six years writing a book which investigates a suicide, while during the past eight and a half years I've been fighting to stay alive because my prostate cells *refuse* to commit suicide (which is what healthy cells do)? Is God besotted with irony?

—Gordon Sheppard, a Canadian writer with metastatic prostate cancer, "The Wondrous World of Prostate Cancer," unpublished essay

---

had no progression of their cancer during the four-year follow-up period. Not surprisingly, the men most likely to respond to salvage beam radiation are those who have a low Gleason score, who have a prolonged PSA doubling time, and who began treatment immediately after their PSA rose.[15]

The third type of beam radiation for prostate cancer recurrence is palliative therapy. It is used for cancers that have spread locally or metastasized to bones or other organs. The intent is to shrink the tumor and thereby provide relief of pain. Such radiation is commonly used in the late stages of the cancer.

Hormone therapy and beam radiation are the most commonly used treatments for recurrent prostate cancer. Surgery is little used except in a few centers, because removal of the prostate after beam or seed radiation therapy is technically very difficult and carries a high incidence of incontinence and other side effects. Seed radiation therapy has been tried following beam radiation or cryotherapy failure, but the results have not been promising. Cryotherapy is sometimes

utilized for recurrent cancer following seed radiation, but its use following beam radiation or surgery has not been encouraging. In assessing all these secondary treatments, we need to carefully weigh
possible benefits against the virtually certain serious side effects.

Chemotherapy is often tried in the late stages of recurrent prostate cancer but with limited benefit. It is relatively ineffective for
prostate cancer, in contrast to many other human cancers. Chemotherapy works best on cancer cells that are dividing very rapidly, and
prostate cancer cells divide slowly compared to other cancers.

The most promising chemotherapeutic regimen for prostate cancer to date has been docetaxel (Taxotere), a drug that has been used
to treat breast cancer, in combination with estramustine (Emcyt) or
prednisone. In late 2004 these combinations were shown in clinical trials to lengthen the life of men with advanced prostate cancer
by approximately two months.[16] This was the first time that any
chemotherapeutic agents had been demonstrated to have an effect
on prostate cancer survival. Many other drugs are being tested, including etoposide (VePesid), mitoxantrone (Novantrone), paclitaxol
(Taxol), carboplatin (Paraplatin), and vinblastine (Velban). Generally these drugs are used in combination with each other or with
hormone therapy.

Chemotherapeutic agents do have significant side effects: hair
loss; fatigue; nausea and vomiting; bone marrow suppression, causing anemia and increased susceptibility to infection; and allergic reactions. Estramustine, one of the most widely used drugs, can also
cause blood clots, which can be fatal. Most of these drugs must be
given intravenously every three to six weeks.

Some men with advanced prostate cancer decide to enroll in
clinical trials of experimental drugs other than chemotherapeutic
agents. Such trials are usually carried out at university medical centers in three phases: phase I assesses whether the drug is safe to be
given to humans, phase II assesses its efficacy dose in a few men, and
phase III tests its efficacy in a large number of men.

Among the most promising ongoing clinical trials are those testing vaccines that tell the body's immune system to attack the cancer.
In 2005 the results of a trial of one vaccine, Provenge, appeared to be
moderately hopeful. Other drugs being studied are those that inhibit
growth factors, cut off the cancer's blood supply (angiogenesis inhib-

itors), promote the death of cancer cells (apoptosis), and inhibit specific enzymes needed by the cancer cells (for example, cyclooxygenase inhibitors such as COX-2).[17] The best way for men to stay current on these studies is by perusing the websites recommended in Appendix C, especially those marked with asterisks.

It has proven to be relatively difficult to persuade men with advanced prostate cancer to enroll in clinical trials. It was estimated in 2003 that four times more women (34,757) were enrolled in breast cancer trials than men (8,309) in prostate cancer trials.[18] A major reason is that most men with advanced prostate cancer are older than most women with advanced breast cancer, and they are not as willing to try to extend their lives for a few additional months. Such trials, however, are essential to finding new and better treatments. Men who wish to identify ongoing clinical trials for which they may be eligible can do so by going to the website of the National Cancer Institute (www.cancer.gov) and clicking on "Clinical Trials." They can also access this information directly by going to a website developed by the National Library of Medicine, www.clinicaltrials.gov (type in "Prostate Cancer" and your city). Another source of information on clinical trials is a commercial website, www.centerwatch .com, which includes a list of drug trials being sponsored by pharmaceutical companies (click on "Oncology," then on "Prostate Cancer").

WEIGHING QUANTITY VERSUS QUALITY OF LIFE

Prostate cancer has the reputation of being a slow-growing and indolent form of cancer. An oft-repeated saying is that many more men die *with* prostate cancer than die *from* prostate cancer. For every hundred men diagnosed with prostate cancer this year, only thirteen will die. We are lulled into thinking of prostate cancer as a rather benign male rite of passage into old age. Fortunately, for the majority of men, it is.

But for a minority of men who get prostate cancer, it is anything but a benign rite. In 2005 it killed more than thirty thousand men in the United States, accounting for 10 percent of all male cancer deaths (second only to lung cancer).

> ### Discussion of Death
>
> Nothing is more inevitable than my death; nothing is more final, irreversible, or irrevocable. For those fortunate enough to have the time to contemplate their own deaths, as I have, nothing is more preoccupying. Very few people seem willing to discuss or even think about these things. "Morbid," they say, as they change the subject. It hasn't been my good fortune to find others willing to share their thoughts and feelings about their own deaths.
>
> —Chuck Wheeler, *Affirming the Darkness*

Prostate cancer deaths are usually not pleasant deaths. Metastases of the cancer to bones can cause bone pain that may become severe and is often worse at night. Fractures of bones secondary to the metastases are not uncommon; if the fractured bone is a vertebra, it may cause compression of the spinal cord, a true medical emergency. The enlarging cancer may also block the urethra or the ureters, producing kidney failure. Weight loss, anemia, and extreme fatigue are common. Studies of men with prostate cancer in the last year of life have reported a slow but steady decline in the quality of life throughout the entire twelve months.[19]

Men who have derived as much benefit as they are likely to get from the multiple forms of prostate cancer treatment should address four tasks. The first is to put their business affairs in order, including writing or updating a will, drawing up a living will in case they become mentally incapacitated, and perhaps designating someone to have power of attorney.

The second task is to thoroughly discuss the issue of pain control with their physicians. Undermedicating patients with advanced cancer has been a severe problem in the United States. Opiates, nerve blocks, and spot beam radiation to treat bone metastases should be readily available for the relief of pain. Injections of strontium-89

Developing a Style

When you're ill you instinctively fear a diminishment and dis-figurement of yourself. It's that, more than dying, that fright-ens you. You're going to become a monster. I think you have to develop a style when you're ill to keep from falling out of love with yourself. It's important to stay in love with yourself. That's known as the will to live. And your style is the instru-ment of your vanity. If they can afford it, I think it would be good therapy, good body narcissism, for cancer patients to buy a whole new wardrobe, mostly elegant, casual clothes.

—Anatole Broyard, *Intoxicated by My Illness*

(Metastron), a radioactive isotope that is selectively taken up by cancer cells in bones, can be highly effective in alleviating pain; it takes four to six weeks to take effect, but may provide relief for up to six months. It is crucial to become knowledgeable about pain control *before* you need it and to convey your wishes to your physicians clearly and concisely. If you think they are not hearing you, put your wishes in writing.

The third task is to assess your support network. Studies have shown that married men decline more slowly than unmarried men.[20] Carefully think through the sources of your own physical and moral support. Visiting nurses and hospices can be extremely helpful in this regard and are strongly recommended.

Part of your moral support is being able to discuss death with others, but those closest to you often avoid the subject. Your prostate cancer support group or members of the clergy can often be helpful in this regard, as can books on death and dying. *Death and Dying* by Elisabeth Kubler-Ross, *How We Die* by Sherwin Nuland, and *Final Gifts* by Maggie Callahan and Patricia Kelley are widely used. Books on cancer in general, such as Stephen Hersh's *Beyond Miracles: Living with Cancer,* contain much useful information on the late stages of

---

Dying with Style

In July 2005, James Smith died at age fifty-five of prostate cancer. Since he was a devout Pittsburgh Steelers football fan, the viewing at the funeral home had Smith's body in a recliner in front of a TV that played continuous Steeler highlight films. He was dressed in pajamas and bathrobe in Steelers colors, had a Steeler blanket on his lap, a beer and pack of cigarettes at his side, and had the TV remote in his hand. Smith's sister noted that "it was just like he was at home."

—*Washington Post,* July 7, 2005

---

cancer and dying. The two best books on dying from prostate cancer are Chuck and Martha Wheeler's *Affirming the Darkness* and Anatole Broyard's classic *Intoxicated by My Illness.*

The final task is to carefully weigh the quantity of your remaining months or weeks against their quality. Broyard urged men "to develop a style" when facing death. How people die is their survivors' final memory of them; it has been called "love at last sight."[21] Cornelius Ryan, facing death from prostate cancer, elected to fight it:

I may "have a rendezvous with death at some disputed barricade." The second to last word is important: the word "disputed."

Come tomorrow, every instinct, every nerve, every fiber in my body has now got the message, I hope that even in anesthesia my mind will dispute that barricade. I will even dispute the Man Upstairs about it—if I have to.[22]

Charles Neider, by contrast, chose to accept it:

But I was ready to go, if need be. Only a young man could have written Dylan Thomas's "Rage, rage against the dying of the light." Raging in this context strikes me, at seventy-eight, as graceless. I admire Socrates, who drank his cup of hemlock with style, and

Robert Falcon Scott, who died quietly and bravely in the tent on the vast Ross Ice Shelf in Antarctica.[23]

It is not important *what* style you choose, merely *that* you choose. For men in whom prostate cancer appears to have won, it is a last chance for both a personal victory and a victory over the cancer.

CHAPTER

12

What Is Known About the Causes?

Once a man has been diagnosed with prostate cancer, he inevitably asks himself: What caused it? Personally, I very much wanted to know. Saying that I had a disease that strikes randomly, like a bolt of lightning, was not very satisfying. It would be better if I could understand its antecedents, even if my own behavior had somehow contributed to its cause.

Yet when I began searching the medical literature for answers, I was disappointed. A 2003 review of the subject stated that "the etiology [cause] of prostate cancer remains virtually unknown."[1] Given that a federal "war on cancer" had been declared in 1971, this assessment was disquieting. Here we are, thirty-five years later, knowing little more than we knew then about the most common cancer to affect American men.

CLUES

In searching for causes of prostate cancer, scientists have major clues to work with. Seven of the most important are the following:

1. *It increases with age.*
   Prostate cancer is the most age-dependent of all human cancers. It is very uncommon in young men; almost three quarters of cases

A Brief History of Prostate Cancer

The first case of prostate cancer in the medical literature was published in London in 1817. Prostate cancer was said to be "a very rare disease" in 1853, and a total of only fifty cases had been described worldwide as late as 1893. During the first half of the twentieth century, the incidence of prostate cancer increased markedly until it became the most common male cancer in Europe and North America. Part of the reason for the dramatic rise is that men are living longer, and prostate cancer increases with age. This accounts for only some of the increase, however; the other reasons are unknown. In recent decades, the incidence appears to have leveled off.

are diagnosed after age 65. However, when prostate tissue is randomly examined from younger men who died from other causes, early subclinical, cancer-like changes, often microscopic in size, are commonly found. In a study of autopsies in Detroit, 30 percent of men in their 30s and 50 percent of men in their 50s showed some early, cancer-like changes in their prostates.[2] So apparently whatever initiates the cancer-causing process does so many years before the cancer manifests itself clinically. This suggestion was strengthened by a 2005 study reporting that a man's PSA level in his 30s predicts his chances of later developing prostate cancer.[3]

2. *Its true incidence in the United States has apparently not changed over the past three decades.*

In the early 1990s, there was great interest in what appeared to be a sharp increase in the incidence of prostate cancer. It is now evident that this apparent spike was due to the increasingly widespread use of the prostate specific antigen (PSA) blood test, introduced in 1986, which was detecting more early cases. Allowing for the increase expected with an aging population, the actual age-corrected incidence of prostate cancer in the United States does not appear to

Table 9. Ethnic Differences in Prostate Cancer in the United States, 2004
(age adjusted per 100,000 population)

	Incidence rate	Death rate
African American	272	73
White	164	30
Hispanic	137	24
Asian American	100	14
Native American	54	22

SOURCE: *Cancer Facts and Figures, 2004* (Atlanta: American Cancer Society, 2004).

have changed in recent decades. This fact suggests that whatever is causing the cancer has not changed either.

3. *There are marked differences in incidence among ethnic groups in the United States.*

Ethnic differences in the incidence of prostate cancer are among the greatest for any form of cancer. The incidence and death rates (mortality) for 1996–2000 are shown in Table 9. Thus, African Americans have an incidence of prostate cancer twice as high as Hispanics and five times as high as Native Americans, although all are minority groups. Minority group status per se does not seem to explain the differences in incidence. The incidence rate for African Americans is 66 percent higher than for whites. The comparable rate for 1973–1977 also shows a 66 percent difference, indicating that the disparity did not change between the 1970s and the 1990s.[4]

Possible reasons for the high incidence of prostate cancer among African American men have been widely debated; suggestions have included genes, diet, and testosterone level.[5] Their high death rate is more understandable, since African American men are less likely to get PSA testing or rectal exams and have less access to specialized medical professionals.[6] However, even when African Americans and white men have equal access to care, as in the Veterans Administration medical system or with prepaid medical plans, studies report that African Americans still go to their physicians with more advanced stages of prostate cancer.[7] Whether this discrepancy is due to a real difference or to a greater reluctance among African Americans to seek appropriate care remains to be ascertained.

The remarkably low rate of prostate cancer among Native

Table 10. Prostate Cancer Death Rates per 100,000 Men
(age adjusted, for the year 2000)

Trinidad and Tobago	32.3
Sweden	27.3
Norway	26.8
Denmark	23.1
Cuba	22.1
Ireland	21.6
New Zealand	21.2
Chile	19.9
France	19.2
United Kingdom	18.5
Germany	18.4
Australia	18.0
United States	17.9
Canada	17.1
Mexico	16.6
Croatia	15.3
Spain	15.0
Greece	10.7
Russia	6.8
Japan	5.5
Kazakhstan	5.2
Turkmenistan	1.8
China	1.0

SOURCE: *Cancer Facts and Figures, 2003* (Atlanta: American Cancer Society, 2004).

Americans—one third the rate of whites and one fifth the rate of African Americans—has received relatively little attention from researchers. The low prostate cancer rate among Alaskan natives has been confirmed in several studies over the past half-century and is supported by reports of very low Arctic-area rates among Inuit men in Greenland and Sami (Lapp) men in northern Norway.[8] Given the unusual diets of these groups, they would seem to be worth investigation by prostate cancer researchers.

4. *There are marked differences in the incidence of prostate cancer in different countries.*

Although access to health care differs among countries, the incidence of prostate cancer varies markedly even among countries with similar access. The highest rates are for Scandinavian countries

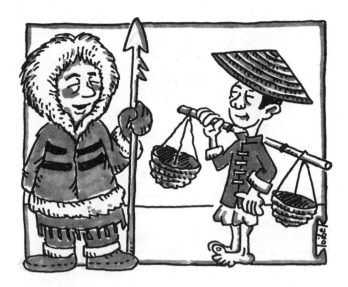

"We must be doing something right!"

(Sweden, Norway, Denmark) and Caribbean countries (Trinidad and Tobago, Cuba). Confirmation of the high rate in the latter came from a study in Jamaica that reported an incidence of prostate cancer among the highest in the world.[9] The high rate of prostate cancer among African Americans and African Caribbeans raises the question of the rate in African nations. A limited number of studies have been done, but those suggest intermediate rates compared to other countries.[10]

At the lower end of the incidence spectrum are countries such as Japan and China, whose rates have been verified in several studies. There is some evidence, however, that the incidence of prostate cancer is increasing in Asia; in both Japan and Singapore, the rate doubled between 1978 and 1997.[11]

In summary, national differences in prostate cancer death rates vary more than thirtyfold. Such massive differences are found in few other diseases except those that are known to be caused by infectious agents.

5. *When men move from a low-incidence country to a high-incidence country, their risk of getting prostate cancer increases.*

Studies of migrants continue to intrigue researchers. Japanese immigrants to the United States have an incidence of prostate cancer four times higher than Japanese men in Japan. Whether the Japanese

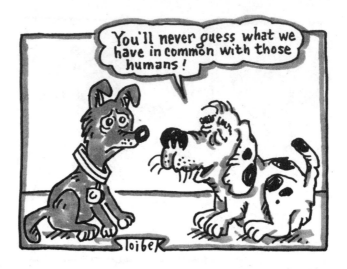

men emigrate to the United States early in life or later in life does not seem to make a difference. Japanese American and Chinese American men who were born in the United States have twice as high an incidence of prostate cancer as Japanese and Chinese men who are immigrants. Similarly, Chinese immigrants to Australia have prostates twice as large, as measured by ultrasound, as those of Chinese men in China.[12]

6. *Dogs are the only mammals besides humans that frequently develop spontaneous prostate cancer.*

Prostate cancer in dogs is similar to that in humans in many ways. It is age dependent and becomes clinically manifest as cancer at a time corresponding to human cancer.[13] Dog prostate glands show similar cancer-like changes in younger dogs. Finally, prostate cancer in dogs has a tendency to spread to lymph nodes and bones, just as it does in humans. One of my colleagues, on reading a draft of this book, asked whether anything is known about the relative incidence of canine prostate cancer in different countries. Alas, the answer is apparently no.

7. *The incidence of prostate cancer among men with schizophrenia is low.*

Five studies of cancer incidence among individuals with schizophrenia in Denmark, Finland, and Israel have reported an unusually low rate of prostate cancer; in the Scandinavian studies, the rate was approximately half the rate expected. A follow-up study suggested that antipsychotic medication may exert a protective effect.[14] Genes, diet, and decreased exposure to other possible causative agents should also be considered.

Given the known facts, what might be causing prostate cancer? In recent years, five major theories have received the most research attention. Let us now consider each of them.

GENES

It is clear that genes play a role in causing prostate cancer, just as they are thought to play a role in causing most other forms of cancer. Family studies, especially of twins, show that if your brother or father (first-degree relatives, who share half your genes) or uncle or grandfather (second-degree relatives, who share a quarter of your genes) had prostate cancer, your chances of getting it are approximately twice as high as if they did not. An affected brother increases your risk a little more than an affected father, and an affected brother or father increases your risk a little more than an affected uncle or grandfather.[15]

If two of your first-degree relatives had prostate cancer, your chances of getting it are five times greater than if none of them had it. If three first-degree relatives had prostate cancer, your chances of getting it are ten times greater. In one family, five out of six brothers developed prostate cancer.[16] Such family clusters are rare, but when they occur, the cancer tends to appear at a young age.

If your family members had cancer in organs other than the prostate, does that increase your risk? Some studies have suggested that having breast or brain cancer in the family increases your risk of prostate cancer, but not all studies agree. The prostate cancer risk appears to be greater if your female relative had the rare, genetic-type breast cancer caused by BRCA genes, which are known to predispose to breast cancer.

Studying cancer in twins is another way to look for genetic clues. Since identical twins share the same genes but fraternal twins share only half their genes, like all other brothers, one would expect prostate cancer to appear in both identical twins more often than in both fraternal twins if genes play a major causative role. And that is what we find. Studies performed in Sweden, Denmark, and Finland, where national twin registries enable such research, show that if the first twin has prostate cancer, the second twin in a fraternal pair will get it 3 percent of the time, but the second twin in an identical pair will get it 18 percent of the time.[17]

These studies show that genes play *some* role in causing prostate cancer. Researchers have tried hard to identify genes that might be involved and have reported suspicious "candidate" genes on almost every chromosome. Examples include the RNASEL gene on chromosome 1, the MSR1 gene on chromosome 8, and the ELAC2 gene on chromosome 17. Evidence linking these specific genes to prostate cancer, however, is still rather weak. Another type of genetic abnormality, the fusion of two genes, was reported in late 2005 to occur in 80 percent of prostate cancers but not in normal prostate tissue; the question remains whether this is a cause of the cancer or an effect.

The latest trend in genetics research is to look at polymorphisms of candidate genes. If a gene were a car, a polymorphism would be a car with a dented fender. It is a particular variant of a gene and helps determine how active the gene is. Polymorphisms may be inherited and have therefore been invoked to try to explain why some ethnic groups are more predisposed than others to prostate cancer. Genes being closely studied for polymorphisms include those regulating testosterone and other androgens that, as will be explained shortly, may play a significant role in prostate cancer. An example of a recently reported gene polymorphism thought to be associated with prostate cancer is the KLF6 gene, which functions to suppress cell growth.

As recently summarized by one researcher, the evidence "points toward a much more complex genetic basis of prostate cancer than initially anticipated."[18] Genes certainly play some role, but the role may be more modest than many researchers originally expected. Some investigators have concluded that only 5 to 10 percent of prostate cancers have a hereditary basis.[19] The fact is that among identical twin pairs, who share the same genes, only one twin gets prostate cancer in the vast majority of cases. And men who migrate from low-risk countries to high-risk countries rapidly increase their risk without changing their genes. Nongenetic factors are obviously very important.

VIRUSES AND OTHER INFECTIOUS AGENTS

The infectious theory of prostate cancer was fashionable twenty years ago, but most contemporary books do not even mention it. The neglect of this line of research is surprising, since approximately 15 percent of all cancers worldwide are caused by infectious agents. For example, *Helicobacter pylori* bacteria is associated with stomach cancer, hepatitis B virus with liver cancer, human papillomavirus with cervical cancer, Epstein-Barr virus with nasopharyngeal cancer, and human T-lymphocyte virus with some leukemias and lymphomas. Prostate cancer is also a type of cancer that increases in incidence in individuals whose immune system is suppressed; this correlation is consistent with an infectious process. Furthermore, when biopsies of prostatic tissue are examined under the microscope, inflammation is frequently present, consistent with infection. For all these reasons, infectious agents should be seriously considered as possible causes of prostate cancer.

The 1970s saw much interest in herpes simplex virus in prostate cancer. In 1973, for example, a research group at the University of Florida reported finding particles of this virus in prostate cancer cells.[20] Subsequent reports have been both positive and negative, with the latter predominating.

Since 2002 there has been a resurgence of interest in viruses as possible causes of prostate cancer. Cytomegalovirus, Epstein-Barr virus, human herpesvirus 8, human endogenous retrovirus E, and human polyomaviruses have all been reported in prostate tissue. It has been said that "the prostate is a complex habitat where mixed infections with oncogenic [cancer causing] DNA viruses frequently occur and [this] opens the discussion to the potential role of these viruses in the cancer of the prostate."[21]

Drawing the most attention as a candidate for causing prostate cancer is the human papillomavirus (HPV). This virus is known to cause many cases of cervical cancer in women as well as some cancers of the penis and rectum in men. To date, more than twenty studies have asked whether HPV causes prostate cancer; the results have been contradictory, with the majority being negative.[22] One difficulty in doing research on this virus, however, is that there are at least one hundred different human subtypes of HPV.

The big problem with research on viruses and other infectious agents is ascertaining cause and effect. Infectious agents can be found in many bodily tissues, but the fact that they are found there does not necessarily mean that they are causing cancer.

SEXUAL ACTIVITY

The idea that prostate cancer may be caused by specific forms of sexual activity has a puritanical appeal, especially for people who believe that sex was bestowed on humankind exclusively for procreation, not recreation. Conversely, the idea that prostate cancer is caused by sexual activity may also appeal to men inclined toward hedonism, cancer thus becoming for them a badge of a life well lived, a paean to Priapus.

The possibility that certain forms of sexual activity may lead to prostate cancer has been downplayed by many. One expert claimed that "there is no good reason to believe that having an active sex life could stimulate the prostate to grow, or cause prostate cancer."[23] Another wrote that "studies attempting to demonstrate a link between prostate cancer and various sexual issues have universally struck out."[24] These conclusions are surprising, given the number of studies that have reported associations between specific sexual activities and the development of prostate cancer.

One example is sexually transmitted diseases. Between 1971 and 2000, thirty-eight studies on STDs and prostate cancer were published. One summary of this research concluded that "the data suggest an elevated relative risk of prostate cancer among men with a history of sexually transmitted infections." Another reasoned that "the available epidemiological evidence does support a possible link between STDs and prostate cancer." Some of the studies reported having had sex with prostitutes as a risk factor. Others focused on the lifetime number of female sexual partners. For example, a study of 753 men with prostate cancer in Seattle reported that "risk estimates increased directly with a lifetime number of female sexual partners"; men with fifteen or more partners lifetime had approximately twice the risk of developing prostate cancer as men with only one partner.[25]

Not all studies have, however, confirmed these results, and some contradict each other. Some report an early age of first intercourse to

I Wouldn't Change a Thing

It's not unnatural for the patient to think that it's sex that is killing him and to go back over his amatory history for clues. And of course this is splendid material for speculation, both lyrical and ironical. I'm tempted to single out particular women and particular practices that strike me now as more likely to be carcinogenic than others. Coitus interruptus, which was widely practiced before the Pill, seems a likely suspect, and oral sex comes to mind as putting greater strain on the prostate. But after saying this, I want to make clear that I certainly don't hold my cancer against these women— whatever I did, it was worth it. I have no complaints in that direction. I wouldn't change a thing, even if I had known what was coming.

—Anatole Broyard, *Intoxicated by My Illness*

be a risk factor, similar to the findings for cervical cancer in women, but other studies do not corroborate this. Nor do researchers agree on what should be measured: frequency of intercourse? frequency of ejaculation? frequency of sex in specific age periods? number of partners? number of extramarital affairs? episodes of STDs in the man? STDs in the partners? exposure to prostitutes? use of condoms?

A possible problem is bias in data collection: Do men with prostate cancer exaggerate their sexual activity when asked about it retrospectively, after they have been diagnosed with cancer? A 2005 study of this question reported that men do not exaggerate the age of their first sexual activity or the lifetime number of their sexual partners.[26] Another problem has been reliance on a single study of Catholic priests that reported their prostate cancer rate to be slightly higher than that of nonpriest controls.[27] Under the assumption that priests are celibate, this study has been widely cited as having proven that sexual activity is not a cause of prostate cancer.

There are ways around these methodology problems. For

example, in one study showing that having had syphilis or gonor-
rhea increased chances of getting prostate cancer, researchers also
collected blood specimens from the subjects and confirmed their
history of syphilis by measuring antibodies in the blood.

HORMONES

In 1941 Charles Huggins demonstrated that blocking the production
of testosterone slows the growth of prostate cancer (as discussed in
Chapter 5). Sixty-five years after Huggins' findings, we are not much
further ahead; we are still blocking testosterone to slow the growth of
prostate cancer, especially in cases when the cancer has spread. Additional evidence that testosterone is involved in causing prostate cancer comes from a variety of sources. Rats given high doses of testosterone develop prostate cancer. Eunuchs and other males who are
castrated prior to puberty do not produce testosterone and do not
develop prostate cancer. Men with cirrhosis of the liver, a condition
that increases their female sex hormone, which suppresses testosterone, have a lower incidence of prostate cancer. The cumulative evidence strongly suggests a role for testosterone.

Although testosterone, made largely by the testes, is the most
important of the male sex hormones (called androgens), it is metabolized in the prostate to dihydrotestosterone (DHT) by an enzyme.
The further metabolism of testosterone and DHT within the prostate
is complex and involves several other androgens, enzymes, and re-
ceptors. The eventual product is the activation of genes, protein syn-
thesis, and proliferation of cells in the prostate. This process can go
wrong at many places, possibly resulting in prostate cancer.

At least twelve studies have measured testosterone and DHT in
individuals with prostate cancer, but only one "was able to show
definitely that men with higher serum levels of testosterone have a
higher risk of prostate cancer."[28] Among the many problems with
these studies is that we do not yet know which androgen, enzyme, or
receptor is the crucial one to measure. Another difficulty is that measuring these hormones in a person's blood may not accurately reflect
what is going on in the prostate. The timing of the blood draw is also
important; serum levels of testosterone vary during the day from a
peak in the morning, when libido is usually highest, to a low point in

the evening. In addition, serum testosterone levels may be affected by surgery, stress, and diet; for example, a high-fat diet increases testosterone.

Most important, we know that prostate cancer begins many years before it is detected, so the critical hormonal changes may take place many years before they are measured, perhaps during puberty. It has even been speculated that prostate cancer begins during the prenatal development of the prostate. If, indeed, the critical hormonal events causing prostate cancer occur during adolescence or earlier, measuring hormones forty or more years later is unlikely to provide definitive answers.

It has been questioned whether differences in male hormones may explain the ethnic differences in the incidence of prostate cancer. In one study of 525 blacks and 3,654 whites, the testosterone levels among blacks were 3 percent higher. A study of Japanese men, who have a low incidence of prostate cancer, found a comparatively low level of DHT and of the enzyme that converts testosterone to DHT. Other studies have reported virtually no differences in testosterone or associated androgens among ethnic groups.[29] It thus remains to be seen whether ethnic differences in hormones are real and, if so, whether they are related to ethnic differences in prostate cancer.

DIETARY FACTORS

Studies on fats and other dietary factors as possible causes of prostate cancer have been ongoing for over thirty years. Currently such theories are fashionable, with one author declaring flatly that prostate cancer "is an apparent casualty of the sedentary Western lifestyle and its notoriously unhealthy diet—rich in animal fat, processed fare, fast and other junk food, and poor in fresh vegetables and fruits."[30] A major impetus behind dietary theories of prostate cancer is the fact that migrants from low-risk to high-risk countries, as from Japan to the United States, rapidly increase their incidence of prostate cancer; it has been speculated that this is most likely a result of their changed diet.

The primary evidence used to link fat intake to prostate cancer is studies showing that countries in which people eat large amounts of

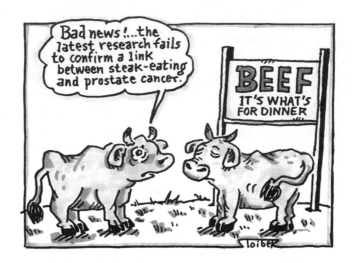

fats are also countries with high rates of prostate cancer. In one study of thirty-two countries, for example, the authors concluded that "mortality from cancer of the prostate is highly correlated with total fat consumption."[31]

To date, at least forty retrospective studies have been done on fat intake and prostate cancer. Some have examined subtypes of fat, such as saturated, monounsaturated, and polyunsaturated. Others have taken into account the source of the fat, such as meat, dairy products, and eggs. The geographical association studies, such as those described above, have been remarkably consistent in showing an association between total fat intake and prostate cancer—with some notable exceptions. Eskimos, for example, have a very high fat intake but a low incidence of prostate cancer.

On the other hand, prospective studies, in which dietary information is collected and the subjects are then followed to ascertain the incidence of prostate cancer, have almost all been negative. In a Norwegian study of 25,708 men followed for more than ten years after dietary information had been collected, "no association was found between energy-adjusted intake of total fat, saturated fat, mono-unsaturated fat, or poly-unsaturated fat and incidence of prostate cancer." For such reasons, according to experts in this field, the "fat-cancer association [has] now become more tenuous."[32]

In addition to fats, excess dietary calcium and zinc have been claimed to promote prostate cancer. In both cases, extremely high quantities were needed to produce the association, and other studies have not confirmed the results. Zinc is of special interest; the prostate, for unknown reasons, contains a higher concentration of zinc than any other organ.

All dietary studies have problems: People do not eat fat, calcium, or zinc alone, but as part of a varied diet containing many foods. Fats may promote cancer not because of their content but rather because of the way the meat is cooked. Fats are also known to increase male sex hormones, so the actual mechanism of cancer enhancement may be hormonal. And perhaps most important, since prostate cancer is thought to begin many years before it becomes manifest, the relevant dietary information may be what the person ate many years earlier.

In addition to dietary factors that may promote prostate cancer, recent attention has focused on foods that may protect against it. The most impressive data have been for tomatoes, on which over a hundred studies have been published. Other dietary factors under study include green tea, red wine, soybeans, yellow and green vegetables, fiber, vitamin A, vitamin D, vitamin E, and selenium (see Chapter 13).

OTHER POSSIBILITIES

The five factors discussed above are the leading candidates as contributors to the causation of prostate cancer. A multitude of other factors have been investigated, but none appear to be as promising. The most serious attention has been given to smoking, alcohol, vasectomy, and exposure to dioxin or cadmium.

Smoking. Since smoking is a known risk factor for lung and bladder cancers, it has been extensively studied for other cancers as well. At least sixty-five research groups have examined smoking and prostate cancer, with the majority reporting no relationship.[33] Men who smoke are more likely to consume a high-fat diet, which may explain research that has found a relationship. A few studies suggest that smoking hastens the spread of prostate cancer once it develops, but other studies have not confirmed this.

Alcohol. Heavy alcohol use is associated with cancers of the liver, larynx, and esophagus. At least thirty-five studies have examined alcohol use and prostate cancer. The conclusion of one review was that "moderate alcohol consumption up to about three drinks per day does not appear to influence prostate cancer risk."[34] Equivocal support was found for the possibility that heavy alcohol use (eight or more drinks a day) may increase the risk. On the other hand, two studies of autopsy tissue taken from men who died from cirrhosis of the liver reported fewer instances of prostate cancer than expected. Cirrhosis increases the production of estrogens, which block testosterone, and thus slows the growth of prostate cancer. Severe alcoholism may therefore decrease the chances of developing prostate cancer.

Vasectomy. Surgical cutting of the vasa deferentia, the ducts that carry sperm from the testicles, is a common form of male contraception. Studies carried out in the 1980s and early 1990s suggested that men who had had a vasectomy, especially if it had been performed when they were relatively young, were at increased risk for prostate cancer. Subsequent studies have refuted this finding; a 1998 review of fourteen studies, for example, concluded that "no causal association was found between vasectomy and prostate cancer."[35] It is now believed that earlier studies did not correct for selection bias; men who had had vasectomies were more likely to go to urologists for follow-up, and urologists in turn would have been more likely to look for prostate cancer in these men.

Dioxin. A component of some herbicides used by farmers and also of Agent Orange, a defoliant used during the Vietnam War, dioxin has been linked to a variety of cancers. Many, but not all, studies of occupational risk exposure have reported that prostate cancer occurs at a disproportionately high rate among farmers. A preliminary study of Vietnam veterans claimed that men with prostate cancer were approximately twice as likely as men without prostate cancer to report having been exposed to Agent Orange.[36] A larger confirmatory study is needed.

Cadmium. The fact that asbestos causes mesothelioma, a form of cancer, has led to a suspicion that industrial carcinogens may cause other cancers. In addition, feeding various chemicals to rats can produce prostate cancer in them. In 1965 it was reported that an excess number of cases of prostate cancer had occurred in a factory where workers were exposed to cadmium. This finding was especially interesting since cadmium inhibits zinc, which is in high concentration in the prostate. Extensive studies have subsequently been carried out on the incidence of prostate cancer among workers exposed to cadmium with the conclusion that there is "no indication for an increased risk of prostate cancer" among the workers.[37]

SUMMARY OF CAUSES

Despite having spent almost $200 billion since 1971 for a "war on cancer," we know little more about the causes of prostate cancer now than when "war" was declared. At least seven clues should help direct our research.

1 Prostate cancer is found predominantly in older men.
2 Its incidence in the United States has apparently not changed in recent decades.
3 There are marked ethnic differences in incidence and death rates in the United States, with the rates for African Americans being high, for whites and Hispanics intermediate, and for Asian Americans and especially Native Americans low.
4 The incidence is very high in Scandinavian and Caribbean nations and very low in Asian nations; the United States is intermediate.
5 Men who migrate from low-incidence to high-incidence countries rapidly acquire the higher prevalence of their new country.
6 Other than humans, dogs are the only mammals that frequently get prostate cancer.
7 The incidence of prostate cancer among men with schizophrenia is low.

Genes play some role in causing prostate cancer, as indeed they do in causing most cancers and most chronic diseases. However, it does not appear that a man inherits genes that directly *cause* the cancer; rather, it seems likely that he inherits several genes that make it more likely that he will get cancer if he is exposed to a factor or factors whose identity is still unknown. Such genes are called *predisposing* genes.

Infectious agents should be carefully studied as possible causes of prostate cancer. To date, several suspects have been brought in for questioning but were released owing to lack of firm evidence. They continue to be under suspicion. Similarly, some aspects of sexual activity appear to play a role in causing prostate cancer, perhaps through having more sexual partners or increased exposure to sexually transmitted diseases.

Male sex hormones undoubtedly play a part in causing prostate cancer, but their specific role is uncertain. The hormonal changes could be a primary cause of the cancer or a secondary effect of diet, infectious agents, or other primary causes. Excess dietary fat has been extensively investigated as a cause of prostate cancer; recent studies suggest that it is a less likely trigger than previously believed. Excess calcium and zinc have also been studied as risk factors, with inconclusive results.

It is likely that some of these factors interact with others. For example, both dietary factors and infectious agents may affect male hormones, which in turn may increase sexual activity and result in sexually transmitted diseases that affect the prostate. In a genetically predisposed individual, such infections may result in cancer.

The biggest impediment to discovering the causes of prostate cancer is that the important events may occur early in life, even decades before the cancer becomes manifest.

13

Factors That May Prevent
Emergence or Recurrence

Given that one in every six American men is expected to be diagnosed with prostate cancer during his lifetime, we might anticipate that major research would have been undertaken to prevent its emergence or recurrence. The National Cancer Institute and other research groups neglected prevention research for so many years that today we know remarkably little. Most prostate cancer prevention trials were initiated only within the past five years and will therefore not yield useful data for many years to come. For example, trials of selenium and vitamin E (the SELECT trial); beta-carotene and vitamins C and E (Physicians Health Study II); and the anti-inflammatory drug rofecoxib will not be completed until 2012 or later.

Theories about the prevention of prostate cancer and its recurrence fall into four categories: they are based on dietary factors, vitamins and minerals, medications, and lifestyle changes. Except for the first of these, remarkably few hard data are available to help men make decisions about what to do. Indeed, in relatively few major diseases do anecdotal data and personal opinions so outweigh factual data. The prevention of prostate cancer is a subject that generates far more heat than light.

DIETARY FACTORS

Dietary factors have been linked to prostate cancer, both as possible causes of the disease and as ways to prevent its emergence or recurrence. Red meat, fat, and excessive zinc are examples of dietary items that are possible causes, as discussed in Chapter 12; reducing your intake of such items may reduce your chances of getting prostate cancer.

Dietary factors linked to possible prevention are in a different category. These food items are not thought to *cause* the cancer but rather to possibly *prevent* its emergence or continued growth. Many authors, in discussing dietary factors, confuse cause and prevention, writing as if the failure to consume sufficient preventive dietary items, such as soy and green tea, causes prostate cancer. This is almost certainly not true; most Inuit Eskimos, for example, do not eat soy or drink green tea and yet have a very low incidence of prostate cancer.

The dietary factors that have been mentioned most prominently as possibly having a preventive action against prostate cancer include the following:

Tomatoes

The best evidence for a food that may slow the development of prostate cancer is available for tomatoes. Among sixteen studies carried out to ascertain the relationship between tomato intake and reduced prostate cancer, six found a significant relationship, three found a trend that was not statistically significant, and seven reported no relationship. In a study of 47,000 health professionals, men who consumed "more than 10 half-cup servings of tomato products per week had a 35% lower risk of developing prostate cancer compared to men who never ate tomato products." Similarly, among 14,000 Seventh Day Adventist households, men "consuming more than 5 servings of tomatoes per week had a 43% lower risk of prostate cancer compared to men who ate less than 1 serving of tomato products per week." Also impressive are two studies in which men ate large amounts of tomato products in the weeks between being diagnosed with prostate cancer and having their prostates surgically removed; in both studies their PSA levels declined.[1]

John Kerry's Diet

Following Senator John Kerry's diagnosis of prostate cancer and surgery in 2002, his wife, Teresa, persuaded him to
change his diet. According to one account: "She has worked
hard, she said, to educate her husband 'to eat smart'—and to
break him of his habit of eating pasta, ice cream, and 'bags of
chocolate chip cookies from the Faneuil Hall market in Boston
that are full of butter.'

" 'He always did eat salad, but he wouldn't eat cooked
greens,' she said. 'Now he always has broccoli and loves brussels sprouts.' He also eats more salads and tomatoes, green
peas, lentils, beans and other vegetables, she said."

—L. K. Altman, *New York Times,*
October 3, 2004

What is not known is the ingredient in tomatoes that is responsible for this apparent effect. It has been widely assumed to be lycopene, a plant carotenoid abundantly present in tomatoes, but in
one animal study, tomato powder was more effective than purified
lycopene in shrinking the tumors.[2] Studies also suggest that tomato
sauce, paste, or cooked tomatoes are more effective as anticancer
agents than are raw tomatoes.

One should not invest heavily in tomato-farm stocks yet, however. Dietary studies are notoriously difficult to carry out because
people do not accurately recall what they ate in the past. More serious
is that dietary information in most studies is gathered for men in
middle and old age, when in fact the critical dietary intake for prostate cancer development may occur much earlier in life. In addition,
Americans are said to consume an average of ninety-one pounds
of tomatoes per year, mostly as pasta sauce, ketchup, pizza, chili,
and salsa. If tomatoes are truly effective in preventing prostate cancer, why is the disease so prevalent? Because of such problems, the
Food and Drug Administration in late 2005 rejected a request by

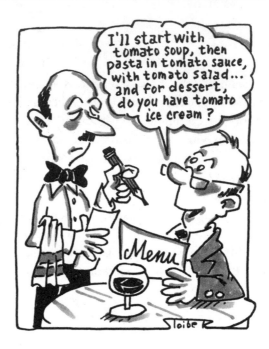

tomato product manufacturers to advertise their products as having cancer-related benefits.

Green Tea

Indigenous to Southeast Asia, tea was introduced into Europe and America in the seventeenth century. Other than water, it became the most widely consumed beverage in the world; it played a significant role in the American Revolution, and its importation made a few men, including John Jacob Astor, wealthy. Worldwide, the drinking of black tea (80 percent) far outstrips that of green tea (20 percent), but in China the percentages are reversed. Green tea is made in such a way that the chemical composition essentially remains similar to that of fresh leaves, whereas black tea has a somewhat different chemical composition.

Except for tomatoes, the evidence to support green tea as possibly preventing prostate cancer is stronger than for any other dietary factor. In animal studies, green tea has been shown both to prevent artificially induced prostate cancer and to reduce the size of existing cancers. The extremely low incidence of prostate cancer in China, where green tea is drunk in large quantities, has led many to suspect a direct relationship between these two facts. In Zhejiang Province, where green tea is widely grown, it "is typically the only non-alcoholic beverage consumed by men, especially older men, throughout their lifetime." Patients with prostate cancer were compared to patients with other diseases on the frequency, duration, and quantity of green tea consumption. More controls than prostate cancer patients were green tea drinkers (80 percent versus 55 percent); the controls also drank more tea and had been drinking it for more years. Drinking fresh tea was especially important, so that "increasing the number of new batches brewed per day to 2 or more was associated with a 76% reduced risk of cancer."[3] Despite such studies, in 2005 the Food and Drug Administration denied requests to label green tea as an effective cancer prevention agent.

It is uncertain what ingredient of green tea is responsible for its possible effect on prostate cancer. Many researchers suspect it is the polyphenols, which have been shown to have antioxidant properties and also to decrease the levels of androgens. Studies suggest that black tea, the kind widely consumed in America and Europe, offers some degree of prostate cancer prevention, but not as much as green tea.

Soy

Soybeans are indigenous to Southeast Asia and consumed extensively in Japan and Korea, mostly as tofu (bean curd), natto (fermented soybeans), and soymilk. Soybeans contain estrogen-like compounds called flavonoids, one of which, isoflavone, is thought to have anticancer properties.

Soy products may also be preventive agents, because until recently prostate cancer was rare in Japan. It is interesting that the incidence of prostate cancer increases sharply among Japanese men who migrate to the United States, where they presumably eat a modified diet that, among other factors, includes less soy.

Isoflavones have been studied in animal models of prostate cancer with mixed results. In some but not all studies, isoflavones appeared to decrease the onset of cancer or reduce the size of existing

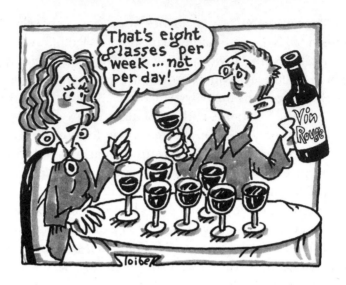

cancers. Most human studies in which soy intake was compared for patients with prostate cancer and for controls have shown little or no difference; one study published in 2004 did show a statistical difference for the consumption of tofu and natto.[4] If soy products do have an effect on prostate cancer, it may be because of their estrogen-like properties, which would block testosterone.

Red Wine and Red Grapes

There are suggestions that red wine and red grapes may provide some protection against prostate cancer. A study conducted in Seattle compared 753 men with prostate cancer to 703 matched controls. In an extensive dietary survey, the controls were found to have consumed more red wine but not white wine, beer, or liquor. For each glass of red wine consumed per week, there was a 6 percent reduction in risk for prostate cancer. According to the researchers, "consumption of 8 glasses or more of red wine per week significantly reduced the relative risk of more aggressive prostate cancer by 61%."[5] Like soy, red wine contains flavonoids that may exert an anticancer effect through their estrogen-like properties. Red grapes contain resveratrol, a compound closely related to flavonoids that also has antioxidant and anti-inflammatory properties. These studies should be confirmed before men make major changes in their alcohol intake.

Michael Milken's Diet

Michael Milken was a prominent Wall Street financier who was imprisoned for securities fraud in the 1980s. After his release, he was diagnosed in 1993 with prostate cancer that had spread to his lymph nodes. He had hormone therapy and radiation, and began a strict diet—extremely low fat and containing large quantities of soy, tofu, green tea, antioxidants, and vitamin E. According to one account: "A typical lunch, prepared by his private dietitian, consists of mushroom barley soup, a tofu egg-salad sandwich (the 'egg' is actually tofu with mustard and spices) with carrots and lettuce, and a black-bean-and-corn salad with a soy-based drink. One of Milken's favorites, an Egg McNothing, consists of a fat-free crumpet with soy cheese, vegetarian Canadian bacon and scrambled egg whites." Milken and his chef have even published *The Taste of Living Cookbook,* specifically for men with prostate cancer.

In addition to his diet, Milken uses meditation, yoga, sesame-oil massages, and aromatherapy to stimulate his immune system. Twelve years after being diagnosed, Milken continues to work and do well. Few men, however, would be willing to follow such a diet and regimen, and almost none have their own personal dietitian and chef.

—Leon Jaroff, "The man's cancer,"
Time, April 1, 1996

Other

A single study of 1,294 men with prostate cancer and 1,451 men without cancer reported that the controls had consumed significantly more vegetable, but not fruit or cereal, fiber.[6] Dietary fiber has been identified as a possible protective factor for other forms of cancer, specifically colon, breast, and ovarian.

Vegetables such as cabbage, cauliflower, turnips, broccoli, kale, and brussels sprouts were linked to the prevention of prostate cancer in one study.[7]

The effectiveness of dietary approaches in preventing the emergence or recurrence of prostate cancer is still to be determined. Each man has to decide what trade-offs he is willing to make, weighing the importance of giving up foods he really likes and eating more of some foods he does not like. What for one man is a sensible, healthy diet may for another man be dietary masochism.

VITAMINS AND MINERALS

Vitamins and minerals have attracted much attention as possible preventive factors for prostate cancer, with many websites featuring them prominently. But anecdotes heavily outweigh facts. The vitamins and minerals that have been most studied in relation to the prevention of prostate cancer are selenium, vitamin E, vitamin A, beta-carotene, and vitamin D.

• *Selenium.* Selenium is a trace metal and a necessary component of several enzymes, especially one (glutathione peroxidase) thought to prevent free-radical damage to cell structures. Selenium is thought to work closely with vitamin E and is theorized to have antioxidant properties, enhance immune function, and decrease testosterone. A longitudinal study of aging men in Baltimore reported that men with lower levels of blood selenium were more likely than others to develop prostate cancer. In contradiction, however, the area of the world where men are most likely to be selenium deficient is China, where the incidence of prostate cancer is very low. A large study (SELECT: the Selenium and Vitamin E Cancer Prevention Trial) is under way to assess selenium and vitamin E as preventive factors for prostate cancer, but the results will not be known until 2013.

• *Vitamin E.* The main component of vitamin E is alpha-tocopherol, which is believed to be an antioxidant that works in conjunction with selenium. Vitamin E was previously thought to help prevent heart attacks, but this property is now in question; one study even concluded that high doses of vitamin E may increase heart attacks. A study in Finland in which men who were smokers were given alpha-tocopherol to see if it would prevent lung cancer found no effect on lung cancer but a 32 percent reduction in prostate cancer. Other studies of vitamin E and prostate cancer have yielded highly conflicting results.[8] Fifteen thousand physicians are being studied in the United States to assess the effects of vitamins E and C and beta-carotene on the incidence of prostate cancer, but the results will not be available until 2012.

• *Vitamin A and beta-carotene.* Vitamin A is essential for cells in the eye having to do with vision. A precursor of vitamin A, beta-carotene is metabolized to a compound that functions as vitamin A. Beta-carotene is closely related to lycopene, the ingredient in tomatoes thought to be responsible for their prostate-cancer preventive effect. Studies linking vitamin A and beta-carotene with prostate cancer have been contradictory, with some reporting a preventive effect and others claiming an increase in the incidence of prostate cancer. A trial of beta-carotene to prevent lung cancer resulted in an *increase* in lung cancer; in recent years interest in these compounds as cancer preventive agents has markedly decreased.[9]

• *Vitamin D.* Formed in the skin by exposure to sunlight, vitamin D is essential for bone formation. Interest in vitamin D and prostate cancer arises from epidemiological observations that prostate cancer is, with some exceptions, more prevalent in northern-latitude nations that get less sunlight and among persons with dark skin that absorbs less sunlight. One study reported that high-dose calcitriol, a form of vitamin D, decreased PSA levels in patients with advanced prostate cancer.[10] Additional trials are in progress.

MEDICATIONS

The idea that specific medications may prevent the emergence or recurrence of prostate cancer arose primarily from observations on finasteride (Proscar). This substance blocks the enzyme that converts testosterone to dihydrotestosterone (DHT), thereby reducing the size of the prostate. It has proven especially effective as a treatment for benign prostatic hypertrophy (BPH).

A trial of finasteride in the prevention of prostate cancer began in 1993 with over eighteen thousand men (Prostate Cancer Prevention Trial). The results, published in 2004, showed that finasteride "did

Caution: The Molière Principle

Molière, the seventeenth-century French playwright, once wrote: "Nearly all men die of their remedies, and not of their illnesses." This principle is important to remember when attempting to prevent prostate cancer. Excessive consumption of selenium may produce abdominal pain, arthritis, emotional instability, hair loss, and liver dysfunction. Excessive consumption of vitamin E may increase a bleeding tendency and the incidence of strokes. Excessive consumption of vitamin D may produce kidney damage, and excessive exposure to sunlight as a way of increasing vitamin D absorption may lead to skin cancers. Excessive consumption of vitamin A may produce hair loss, elevated blood lipid levels, neurological symptoms, and liver damage.

indeed significantly reduce the prevalence of prostate cancer but did so at a disturbing price: the possibility that if cancer is detected, it may be of a higher pathological grade."[11] The reduction in prostate cancer was 25 percent, but this good news was offset by the bad news that the cancers that did occur were more malignant than expected. Thus, it is not recommended that finasteride be used to prevent prostate cancer.

Tests of other medications to reduce prostate cancer are in progress, including a trial of dutasteride, a drug similar to finasteride, in eight thousand men (the REDUCE study). Statins, used to lower cholesterol, have shown some promise; one study reported that statin use decreased PSA, and another found that it decreased the incidence of prostate cancer. However, in 2006 a large study of statins concluded that they had no effect on any cancers, including cancer of the prostate.[12] Also being investigated are drugs that decrease inflammation; studies of long-term aspirin users suggest that aspirin may lower the risk of developing prostate cancer.[13] A study of rofecoxib (Vioxx), a cyclooxygenase (COX-2) inhibitor, was under way until the drug was withdrawn in 2004 because of its cardiac side effects. Research on another COX-2 inhibitor, celecoxib (Celebrex), is planned.

LIFESTYLE CHANGES

Lifestyle changes are recommended for the control and prevention of all cancers, including prostate cancer. Like motherhood, these recommendations are hard to disagree with.

The relationship between physical activity and prostate cancer has been examined in at least twenty-eight studies, with inconsistent results. Two reported that physical activity and exercise did not reduce the *incidence* of prostate cancer but reduced the *severity* of the cancer that developed.[14] Weight control is desirable for many reasons, but its effect on prostate cancer is ambiguous. One study reported that obese men were more likely to see progression of their cancers; another study found that cancer was less likely to be detected in obese men because their prostate glands are larger; still another study claimed that middle-aged obese men have a *decreased* risk of prostate cancer.[15] Not smoking and drinking alcohol only in moderation are universally recommended for cancer prevention.

Regarding diet, the American Cancer Society advocates the following steps to reduce the risk of cancer. These guidelines are consistent with recommendations for preventing heart disease, diabetes, and other conditions:

- Eat five or more servings of vegetables and fruits each day.
- Choose whole grains instead of processed (refined) grains and sugars.
- Limit consumption of red meats, especially high-fat and processed meats.
- Choose foods that help maintain a healthful weight.

When diet and lifestyle changes are combined and adhered to faithfully, there is evidence that they may slow the progression of prostate cancer. A controlled study, published in 2005, randomized into two groups ninety-three men who had early-stage prostate cancer and who had elected watchful waiting. The men in one group continued their usual diet and lifestyle. Those in the other group went on a vegan diet with soy, fish oil, selenium, vitamins C and E, exercise, stress management techniques, and a weekly group meeting. At the end of one year, the men on the vegan diet had a 4 percent decrease in their PSA (from an average of 6.23 to 5.98), whereas the diet-as-usual group had a 6 percent increase (from an average of 6.36 to 6.74).[16]

SO WHAT SHOULD YOU DO?

Taking into consideration everything that is known about the emergence and recurrence of prostate cancer, what should you do? Most important, realize that remarkably little is known with certainty, and what is unknown far outweighs what is known. Weigh quantity of life against quality of life. Making some dietary or lifestyle changes after being diagnosed with prostate cancer may not be difficult, whereas you may find making other changes to be quite hard.

I have modified my own diet modestly but not radically. I eat tomatoes in one form or another with each dinner, and I drink tomato juice with lunch. Red grapes are now a staple snack item in our home, always available. I have not given up red meat altogether but have continued to decrease my consumption of it, a trend I had begun several years before being diagnosed with prostate cancer. I increasingly drink green tea and may, if I live long enough, come to like it. I am exploring red wines and have been surprised to discover that many of them, especially the more expensive ones, are very good; my past experience was apparently limited by having bought only inexpensive ones. However, for me they will never completely replace fine Belgian ales or California porters.

I continue to take low-dose aspirin and multivitamins each day, as I had been doing for many years, although I switched from a multivitamin that had supplemental zinc to one without. I stopped taking supplemental vitamin E, based on the most recent cardiac study, and have not started taking supplemental selenium—although I will watch the emerging studies and could be persuaded to do so. Regarding soy and tofu, I draw the line and will wait until I discover a tasty chocolate chip cookie made from soy.

14

Science and Politics

Prostate cancer is a major threat to men's health. Adult men in the United States have a 1 in 6 chance of being diagnosed with it in their lifetime. This compares with a 1 in 13 chance of being diagnosed with lung cancer, 1 in 17 with colon cancer, 1 in 68 with leukemia, and 1 in 81 with stomach cancer. Once diagnosed with prostate cancer, 1 of every 5 men will die from it. In 2005 this translated to an estimated 29,528 deaths, one every eighteen minutes.

Since the American population is aging, the problem will almost certainly worsen. In 2005, approximately 234,000 men were initially diagnosed with prostate cancer; in 2025, the number is projected to be 384,000 men, and in 2045, to be 452,000 men. The projected future costs of prostate cancer are astronomical.

Given these numbers, one might expect that the United States government would long ago have organized a serious effort to uncover the causes of, and better treatments for, prostate cancer. In 1971, in his State of the Union message, President Nixon proposed "an intensive campaign to find a cure for cancer." He affirmed that "the time has come when the same kind of concentrated effort that split the atom and took man to the moon should be turned toward conquering this dread disease." In what subsequently came to be known as the war on cancer, the federal government poured billions of dollars into these efforts, with private industry and donations through organizations such as the American Cancer Society adding more billions. According to a 2004 estimate of cancer research expenditures, "Americans have spent, through taxes, donations, and private R and D [research and development], close to 200 billion, in inflation-adjusted dollars, since 1971."[1]

Prostate cancer has received less than its share of research funds and attention. In the mid-1990s, breast cancer research received approximately seven times more in federal research funds than prostate cancer, despite the fact that approximately the same number of women and men were so diagnosed each year. By 2005 this discrepancy had been reduced, so that breast cancer received approximately twice as much federal funding per diagnosed case.

Prostate cancer research in the United States is supported almost exclusively by three organizations: the National Cancer Institute; the Prostate Cancer Research Program, under the U.S. Department of Defense; and the private Prostate Cancer Foundation, founded by financier Michael Milken.

THE NATIONAL CANCER INSTITUTE

The National Cancer Institute (NCI) is part of the National Institutes of Health (NIH), located in Bethesda, Maryland. Federally funded, its budget for 2006, at more than $5 billion, has doubled since 1997. Despite its massive budget, many have criticized the NCI for the same reasons other NIH institutes have been criticized: the application process for research grants is unnecessarily cumbersome and lengthy; it focuses too much on basic research and not enough on research that is likely to help those who currently have cancer; and it is extremely conservative, so that researchers who are innovative and think outside the box do not get funded. As noted in one analysis of the NCI:

> Somehow, along the way, something important has gotten lost. The search for knowledge has become an end unto itself rather than the means to an end. And the research has become increasingly narrow, so much so that physician-scientists who want to think systemically about cancer or the organism as a whole—or who might have completely new approaches—often can't get funding.[2]

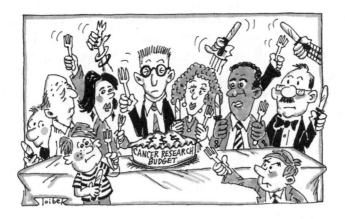

Another shortcoming of the NCI has been its lack of leadership or coordination of cancer research efforts at the national level. Each university and cancer research center gets a piece of the federal budgetary pie and goes off to its own private corner to eat it. Nobody has been putting the pieces together, which has slowed down progress—on prostate cancer as much as on other forms of cancer. Prostate cancer sufferers were hopeful that more progress would be made between 2002 and 2005, when Andrew von Eschenbach was the director of the NCI. He had been diagnosed with prostate cancer and his father had died from it. Changing the course of this federal behemoth, however, proved to be a difficult task.

THE PROSTATE CANCER RESEARCH PROGRAM

The Prostate Cancer Research Program is run by the U.S. Army under the Department of Defense. Its origins are a classic Washington tale.

In 1992, women's advocacy groups for breast cancer research were putting pressure on the federal government to increase funding. Representative Patricia Schroeder, at that time, chaired the House Armed Services Committee, overseeing spending by the Department of Defense. Since expenditures for the National Cancer Institute were restricted by federal regulations, Schroeder arranged to give $25 million to the Army to coordinate additional breast cancer research. Over the next three years, Congress added $390 million more and asked the Institute of Medicine to evaluate the program. The evaluating committee published its report in 1997, calling the Department of Defense breast cancer research "a unique and valuable entity," especially for its "potential to focus on innovation, in ways that go beyond what traditional institutions like the National Institutes of Health are able to do."[3]

Observing the success of the breast cancer lobby, advocates for prostate cancer research decided to follow suit. A dinner was arranged to which, according to one participant, "several members of Congress were invited who just happened to have prostate cancer." In 1997 Congress allocated $45 million to the Department of Defense for what became known as the Prostate Cancer Research Program (PCRP).

Since 1997 Congress has continued to fund this research; in 2006, the allocation was $80 million. Through 2005, a total of over $600 million had been spent on more than fourteen hundred research projects. A prominent part of the program is the Center for Prostate Disease Research, an excellent clinical program for military veterans with prostate cancer directed by Col. David E. McLeod, M.D., at the Walter Reed National Medical Center. Another important component is a tissue bank in which blood and prostate tissue are collected from men with prostate cancer and then made available to researchers. A prostate cancer database registry that includes more than eleven thousand men with prostate cancer is also available to investigators. Whether the Prostate Cancer Research Program will ultimately be any more successful than the National Cancer Institute in funding innovative research or making a major breakthrough on prostate cancer remains to be ascertained, but to date it is well regarded by researchers in this field.

MICHAEL MILKEN'S PROSTATE CANCER FOUNDATION

Michael Milken, a summa cum laude graduate of the University of California at Berkeley and a graduate of the Wharton School of Business, rose to billionaire prominence in the 1980s as the Wall Street "king of junk bonds," high-yield debt securities. Rudy Giuliani, then a New York prosecutor, went after him for securities fraud, and Milken eventually pleaded guilty to six counts of violations related to market manipulation.[4] He paid $600 million in fines and spent twenty-two months in prison. Ironically, both Giuliani and Milken were subsequently diagnosed with prostate cancer and became friends and national advocates for prostate cancer sufferers.

Milken was diagnosed with prostate cancer in 1993, shortly after his release from prison. Just 46 years old, he had a Gleason score of 9, a PSA of 24, and the cancer had already spread to his lymph nodes. He was treated with beam radiation and hormones and began a very strict diet; thirteen years later he remains in remission.

Milken approached prostate cancer in the same manner he had approached Wall Street securities. "I decided that I had to change the course of history," he recalls, and proposed "a Manhattan Project" for prostate cancer to discover the causes and better treatments.[5] He pledged $25 million of his own funds and in 1993 began CaPCURE (cancer of the prostate cure), a foundation that in 2003 was renamed the Prostate Cancer Foundation (PCF).

Milken has accomplished a remarkable amount in pursuit of his goals. Between 1993 and 2003, his foundation raised $230 million and funded over twelve hundred prostate cancer research projects. In contrast to the National Cancer Institute, where getting a research grant funded often takes eighteen months or more, Milken's awards are given in three months. Also in contrast to the NCI, the research projects funded by the foundation are more focused on finding better treatments and less oriented toward basic cellular research.

Milken's foundation has coordinated a prostate tissue bank to distribute tissue to researchers and has set up a genetics project to collect blood from families with three or more members who have prostate cancer. It has also put together a consortium of eight leading prostate cancer research centers and holds an annual meeting to bring leading researchers together to exchange ideas. Perhaps most remarkably, his foundation requires its grantees to cooperate with one another and to openly discuss their research findings, a true accomplishment in a field that has at least its share of prima donnas.

In addition to his research efforts, Milken has attempted to raise the profile of prostate cancer. He has lobbied Congress and worked with other advocacy groups, such as the National Prostate Cancer Coalition, to organize public events. Since 1996 the Prostate Cancer Foundation has worked with major league baseball teams to

> ### A Great Teacher
>
> Cancer is a harsher teacher than inspirational bestsellers or ads for vitamin-mineral supplements. It reminds us that we are *not* immortal, that our time is limited, that disease and death are still out there waiting for us. . . . Cancer is the worm in the apple of jaunty optimism about life; the banana peel on which even the healthiest and fittest of us slips; a great teacher, if you're lucky enough to survive the lesson.
>
> —Michael Korda, *Man to Man*

sponsor a PCF Home Run Challenge that raises public awareness and generates research funds. A laudatory article in *Fortune* in late 2004 concluded that "Milken has, in fact, turned the cancer establishment upside down."[6]

THE NATIONAL PROSTATE CANCER COALITION

The National Prostate Cancer Coalition (NPCC) is the foremost advocacy organization on prostate cancer. It began in 1996, when a group of men who had prostate cancer met in Texas and decided to form an organization modeled after the women's advocacy groups for breast cancer. Mary Lou Wright of the Mathews Foundation for Prostate Cancer Research, a pioneer in the field, was instrumental in getting it started; Michael Milken, the American Cancer Society, and Zeneca Pharmaceuticals (which later became part of AstraZeneca) were also helpful.

Located in Washington, D.C., the NPCC has a staff of twelve and operates with a combination of corporate sponsorship and donations. Its twofold mission is promoting research on, and awareness of, prostate cancer. To accomplish the first, it is active on Capitol Hill and has close relationships with many members of Congress who have prostate cancer—some of whom have publicly acknowledged their illness and others who have not. Senator Ted Stevens of Alaska and former Senator Bob Dole have for many years been the leading congressional voices on prostate cancer.

Both the Senate and the House of Representatives have informal caucuses composed of legislators who have family members with some form of cancer. Members of Congress who have been consistent supporters of prostate cancer research include Senators Michael Crapo (Idaho), Byron Dorgan (N. Dak.), Diane Feinstein (Calif.), Tom Harkin (Iowa), Kay Hutchinson (Tex.), Harry Reid (Nev.), and Jeff Sessions (Ala.), and Representatives Sherrod Brown (Ohio), Lois Capps (Calif.), Jesse Jackson (Ill.), Peter King (N.Y.), Kendrick Meek (Fla.), and Deborah Pryce (Ohio).

In a variety of ways NPCC attempts to increase awareness of prostate cancer, and especially of how important it is that men be tested. It has worked with major league baseball on an education campaign, "Take a Swing Against Prostate Cancer"; with the National Hockey League on a "Hockey Fights Cancer" program; and with NASCAR drivers such as Dale Earnhardt, Jr., and Jimmie Johnson on a "NASCAR Young Guns Consumer Challenge," in which fans can donate at NASCAR races to fight prostate cancer. The NPCC has promoted September as Prostate Cancer Awareness Month, an extension of work by the Prostate Cancer Education Council, a smaller advocacy group in Denver. In many of these activities, NPCC works with other organizations, including Us Too and Milken's Prostate Cancer Foundation.

Much of NPCC's influence comes from "Aware," its free biweekly on-line newsletter, which has over forty-five thousand subscribers. The newsletter includes summaries of breaking news on prostate cancer research and links to the stories. Despite the fact that it carries pharmaceutical company ads and thus cannot be truly objective on drug developments, "Aware" is the most useful and widely read on-line news source for men with prostate cancer.

OTHER PLAYERS

The oldest existing prostate cancer group is the Prostate Cancer Education Council (www.pcaw.com), founded in 1988. It originated

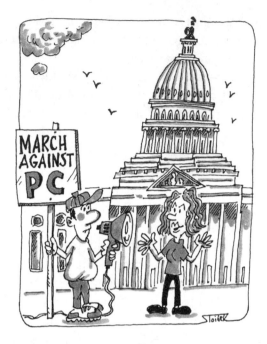

"Like, I totally agree! This 'political correctness'
has gone *waaay* too far!"

Prostate Cancer Awareness Week and has worked hard to make men
aware of the necessity of having regular PSA tests and rectal exams. It
too has corporate sponsorships.

Other cancer organizations serve individuals with all types of
cancer, not just prostate cancer. The largest and oldest is the American Cancer Society (www.cancer.org), which began in 1913. It has
both state and local offices and raises both public awareness and
funds for research and prevention. The National Coalition for Cancer Survivorship (www.canceradvocacy.org), founded in 1986, is the
oldest cancer organization led by cancer survivors themselves. It
works closely with the media to promote education about cancer.
Both of these organizations accept donations.

Finally, there are the pharmaceutical and radiation-related in-
dustries, which stand to gain financially from the widespread use of
hormone and radiation therapies. These companies sponsor prostate
cancer awareness events and cancer screening programs. In late 2004
the Theragenics Corporation, manufacturer of the seeds most com-

monly used for radiation seed therapy, persuaded Congress to pass a resolution "encouraging doctors to inform prostate cancer patients of all the proven treatment options available, including brachytherapy."[7] Congress thereby put itself into the medical information business.

The pharmaceutical industry, however, does not have an especially distinguished record in the prostate cancer field. For example, TAP Pharmaceutics has paid over $1 billion since 2001 to settle a series of civil claims and criminal charges. Jointly owned by Abbott Laboratories and Takeda Chemical Industries, TAP is the manufacturer of leuprolide (Lupron), one of the two major LHRH blockers widely used in hormone therapy. The company was accused of bribing urologists to switch their patients from Zoladex (goserelin) to Lupron. One scheme was to give doctors free Lupron samples and then encourage them to bill Medicare or other third-party payers. In another scheme, "the company gave the federal government an inflated wholesale price for Lupron and then sold the drug to hundreds of doctors at a far lower price. On billing Medicare, the doctors could expect to get $100 or more in illicit profits on every shot."[8] It is alleged that hundreds of urologists cooperated with the company, some netting $30,000 or more.

Has advocacy been effective in raising awareness of prostate cancer and increasing funds for research? It unquestionably has been on both counts. Research funds have increased more than tenfold since 1993. Funds for prostate cancer research, however, still are only approximately half those devoted to breast cancer on a per patient affected or per death basis. Prostate cancer is disadvantaged in its advocacy efforts in that most of those affected are older men, and it is difficult to organize them to march on Congress. Over the last decade prostate cancer, often abbreviated PC, has become somewhat more politically correct, but it still has a long way to go.

CHAPTER

15

Advice for Men Who Do Not Have Prostate Cancer

Chico, one of the comedian Marx Brothers, was once seen by his wife kissing a chorus girl. When pressed for an explanation, he quickly replied: "I wasn't kissing her, I was whispering in her mouth." We men have a remarkable ability to deny the obvious and create excuses—indeed, it may be one of our greatest strengths. Failing to get regular checkups to detect prostate cancer is simply another illustration of "denial vain, and coy excuse," as Milton long ago called it.

SHOULD I BE TESTED?

Many studies of men who have undergone regular exams for prostate cancer, including digital rectal exams and PSA testing, suggest that such precautions save lives. Comparison of 173 men in Minnesota who died of prostate cancer with 346 matched controls reported that only 61 percent of the men who died had had a digital rectal exam in the previous nine years, compared to 81 percent of the men in the control group. The authors of the study concluded that a "screening [exam] may have prevented 50 percent to 70 percent of deaths . . . due to prostate cancer." A study in Washington State of 171 men who died of prostate cancer and 342 matched controls similarly found that "men who have been screened with DRE [digital

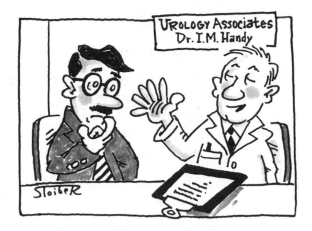

"They say I have a special skill in diagnosing prostate cancer."

rectal exam] and/or PSA are at lower risk of mortality from prostate cancer than men who have not been screened."[1]

The most convincing data, however, come from a study in Austria in which PSA testing was made available without charge to men in one Austrian state but not in others. Within five years, more than two thirds of men aged 45 to 75 in the state with free PSA testing had been tested one or more times. Two years after the study began, the death rate from prostate cancer began falling in that state significantly more than in the other states; the researchers claimed that this trend was "the first evidence . . . that the policy of making PSA testing universally available and at no cost may have led to a reduction in death from prostate cancer in that population."[2]

In contrast to these studies, a highly publicized 2006 study of 501 men who died from prostate cancer in New England reported that screening by PSA or digital rectal exam did not save lives. The authors suggested that physicians should not use the reduction of mortality as a justification for endorsing "routine testing of asymptomatic men." An accompanying editorial, however, noted that 78 percent of male primary-care physicians and 95 percent of male urologists aged 50 and over do have their PSA tested. Two large studies of PSA testing are currently in progress. One, the PLCO Cancer Screening Trial, has registered 74,000 men in the United States; the other, the European Randomized Study of Screening for Prostate Cancer,

PSA Tests as a Godsend

All the debates notwithstanding, PSA tests are a godsend. . . . You should know your PSA number just as you know your cholesterol count. . . . When I sit in meetings at work and look at groups of men who are my contemporaries, I want to shout at them, "Do you guys know what your PSA is?"

—Andy Grove, "Taking on Prostate Cancer,"
Fortune, May 13, 1996

has registered 172,000 men at five European sites.[3] Results of the two studies are expected in 2006 and 2008, respectively. In the meantime, men must decide whether to heed the existing evidence or await definitive results.

Because of such discrepant results, widespread PSA testing continues to be controversial. Some authorities argue that since three quarters of PSAs between 4 and 10 turn out not to be cancer, such testing leads to unnecessary biopsies, expense, and anxiety for the men involved. They point out that PSA testing is not sensitive enough, since it misses 15 percent of men who have significant cancer even though they have PSAs of less than 4. They argue that it has not yet been conclusively proven that PSA testing actually saves lives. Finally, they note that autopsy studies of men dying from other causes have found small foci of prostate cancer in almost all older men, so technically almost all men have some cancer. Opponents of PSA testing received further support in 2004 when Thomas Stamey and his colleagues at Stanford University publicly claimed that "the PSA era is probably over for prostate cancer in the United States."[4]

Predictably, other researchers immediately responded that "the PSA era is not over for prostate cancer."[5] They pointed to data suggesting that PSA screening has been the main reason for the decrease in advanced tumors. For example, between 1983 and 1985, only 75 percent of men diagnosed with prostate cancer were alive five years

---

Kojak's Mistake

Telly Savalas, the bald actor who played the television detective "Kojak," had come in with a PSA of 10, he recalled. "Dr. Skinner scheduled the biopsy, but Savalas had a Christmas special and cancelled it. Then he needed a vacation. I called to tell him how important it was, but he never came back. Four years later he was gone."

—David Horowitz, *The End of Time*

---

later. Between 1995 and 2000, 99 percent of men so diagnosed were alive five years later.

Because of the continuing disagreement about the value of widespread PSA testing, an independent panel of experts was assembled under the Agency for Healthcare Research and Quality. They could not agree either and concluded that "the jury is still out on the value of routine screening" and that "patients should talk with their clinicians to make individualized decisions."[6]

The cycle is complete: men have for years been told that they must make the decision regarding what treatment to pursue if they get prostate cancer. Now, men are also being told that they must make the decision whether even to be tested to determine whether they have prostate cancer. At first glance, it all sounds very democratic, but the truth is that few men have sufficient information to make informed decisions. Is it any wonder that many ignore the whole business and avoid testing altogether, baffled by the plethora of facts and the indecision of experts?

To me it seems self-evident that PSA testing, combined with a digital rectal exam, is not only worthwhile but one of the few things a man can do to diagnose cancer early and possibly save his life. Much of the confusion comes from thinking of PSA testing as either negative (3.9 or lower) or positive (4.0 or higher). We saw in Chapter 2 that PSA is a *continuum* and becomes valuable as a diagnostic tool

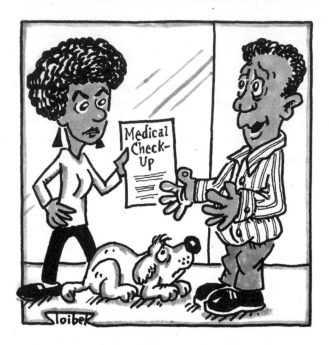

"I think the dog ate my last PSA appointment card."

when measured on a regular basis so that the rate of change (PSA velocity) can be calculated. The argument that almost all older men have microscopic foci of cancer cells in their prostate glands does not negate the value of checking PSA; the testing is an attempt to identify men who have a microscopic focus that, for whatever reason, is growing into a full-blown cancer.

BIOPSIES

If the word *embarrass* was intended to describe any single act, it surely applies to a prostate biopsy. You lie on your side, your backside naked to the world, while your urologist inserts a probe into your rectum, then removes tiny slivers of tissue from your prostate with what sounds like a staple gun. The magnitude of the pain is remarkably minimal compared to the magnitude of the indignity.

When should a man have a biopsy? If your physician feels anything suspicious on digital rectal exam, that is a certain indication.

Surviving a Biopsy

Tying up the gown is the hardest part of the disrobing exercise because it has to be done backwards, and as everybody knows, the "behind-your-back-skills" gene is not carried on the male chromosome the way color-blindness is. Simply put, a man cannot do this task. . . .

Thankfully, I'm facing away from the action, as if I'm on one side of the room, my behind on the other. But from that position I can't watch the monitor with its jerky black and white picture of my prostate, and so can't make futile attempts at humor, which always buoys my spirits and masks my agitation. *Is it a boy or a girl, doctor?*

—Bert Gottlieb, *The Men's Club*

Any significant rise in your PSA level, as defined below, is also an indication.

In preparation for a prostate biopsy most, but not all, urologists ask you to stop taking aspirin compounds a week to ten days prior to the procedure. The night before, you are asked to drink a solution that cleans out your bowel by causing diarrhea. Alternatively, you are also asked to give yourself a Fleet enema prior to the procedure— valuable practice for the humiliation of the biopsy itself.

The urologist first inserts into your rectum the ultrasound probe, equivalent in size to about two fingers. The probe sends out sound waves that outline the prostate on a small screen, allowing the urologist to see exactly where to biopsy. Sometimes the ultrasound shows dark areas that may indicate cancer, but often it fails to show cancer even when it is present. At one time it was hoped that prostate ultrasound would become as useful as the mammography used to detect female breast cancer, but it has proven disappointing for that purpose; its main use is to guide the biopsy and determine prostate volume.

The biopsy itself involves the use of very thin needles that go through the wall of the rectum and into the prostate, where they remove a thin sliver of tissue. Each such piece is called a core. In the past, it was usual to take six cores, but it is now common to take eight to twelve. Lying on the table, you will know exactly how many have been taken by counting the distinctive clicks of the biopsy gun. The pain is a momentary sting, likened by one urologist to "a rubber band being snapped against the skin,"[7] although men vary widely in their pain threshold. The entire procedure takes about a half hour.

Following the biopsy, many urologists have men take an antibiotic for three days to minimize the likelihood of infection. It is normal to have small amounts of blood in the semen, urine, or stool for a few days, and there are no restrictions on activities other than riding a bicycle. Since the biopsy is merely sampling sections of the prostate and not the entire gland, it is possible that cancer is present and is missed by the biopsy. If the urologist is suspicious, if the biopsy shows precancerous cells (prostatic intraepithelial neoplasia, or PIN), or if the PSA continues to rise, the biopsy may have to be repeated at a later date.

In the end, so to speak, the information provided by a prostate biopsy is extremely useful. If the biopsy is negative, the chances are high (approximately 70–80 percent) that cancer is not present. If it is positive, you will know your cell type (Gleason score) and you will also have information on the size of the cancer from the ultrasound picture, the percentage of positive cores, and the percentage of cancer in each positive core. From these you can assess the seriousness of your cancer and begin making rational treatment decisions.

TEN RECOMMENDATIONS

The American Cancer Society currently recommends that men have a digital rectal exam and PSA test annually, beginning at age 50, if they have a life expectancy of at least ten more years. For men who have a family history of prostate cancer and for African American men, with their higher rate of prostate cancer, the recommendation is to begin annual testing at age 45.

Based on a review of the existing literature, my recommendations are as follows. They are based on studies showing that men who

Living with Cancer

Life doesn't end when you have cancer. Instead, it becomes vastly more precious. I find myself reluctant to waste any cherished moment. I will no longer vegetate in front of the TV, as I have in the past. I'm less willing to spend any precious time in anger, argument, long committee meetings, or unnecessary trips.

—Michael Dorso, *Seeds of Hope*

have very low PSA values are unlikely to develop prostate cancer in the immediate future.[8] Knowing what I know now, here is what I personally would do.

1 I would get a baseline PSA by at least age 40 to 45. A 2005 study reporting that a man's PSA level in his 30s predicts the risk of later prostate cancer suggests that getting a baseline PSA even earlier may be useful.[9] If the PSA was less than 1.0, I would not get an additional PSA for five years. If I had a family history of prostate cancer or was African American, I would reduce the interval to two years. As long as my PSA remained less than 1.0, I would continue this practice for successive five-year periods until age 60 unless I developed symptoms of an enlarging prostate.

2 I would get a digital rectal exam each time I had a PSA test.

3 From age 60 on, or if my PSA had risen to between 2.0 and 3.0 before age 60, I would increase the frequency of PSA testing to every year.

4 I would keep a personal record of my PSA test results so that I could assess the PSA velocity. It is one of the most useful predictors of prostate cancer. Knowing your PSA is as important as knowing your cholesterol level.

5 If my PSA rose more than 0.7 in any given year, I would first repeat the test to verify its accuracy. If accurate, I would get a free PSA determination (see Chapter 2), which is a way to identify noncancer

causes of increasing PSA (for instance, prostatitis or benign prostatic hypertrophy).

6 If at any time my PSA indicators were worrisome (PSA velocity greater than 0.7 in a year, free PSA less than 20 percent), I would have a biopsy.

7 If the biopsy turned up any questionable findings, including prostate intraepithelial neoplasia, I would have a repeat biopsy in a few months.

8 If I got to age 75 to 80 without evidence that my PSA was increasing more than the minimal rise expected with age, I would stop having PSA testing.

9 If, at any point, my life expectancy was less than ten more years, I would stop having PSA testing.

10 Even though there is not yet definitive evidence, I would try to modify my diet along the lines recommended in Chapter 13, specifically reducing my fat intake and increasing tomato products, green tea, red wine, and perhaps soy. For most of us, this is much more difficult than undergoing PSA testing and biopsies.

FUTURE RESEARCH

Despite disagreements about the value of PSA screening for prostate cancer, all urologists agree on one fact: We need better tests. The PSA and digital rectal exams are used because they are the best we have; both will be regarded in the future as relatively primitive.

Thanks to the efforts of the advocacy groups and select members of Congress, as described in the previous chapter, research is now under way to design more accurate tests for diagnosing prostate cancer and for identifying which prostate cancers are likely to remain quiescent and which are likely to spread. This research involves proteins found in the blood, proteins found in the prostate tissue, genes, and imaging techniques.

Among the candidates in the blood for predicting prostate cancer are proteins with names such as caveolin–1, insulinlike growth factor binding proteins (IGFBP 2 and 3), interleukin 6 and its receptor (IL–6 and IL6R), kallikrein 2, telemerase, and a transforming growth factor (TGF beta 1). An especially promising approach reported in late 2005 uses several proteins that are part of the immune system's response to cancer; according to the report, "the panel of [proteins] performed better than did prostate-specific antigen (PSA) in distinguishing between the group with prostate cancer and the control group."[10]

Several proteins found in the prostate tissue itself, available by biopsy or surgery, appear promising for predicting the severity of the cancer. These include alpha methylacyl-coenzyme A racemase (AMACR), annexins, Bcl-2 and other factors that control the death of cells (apoptosis), E-cadherin, enhancer of zeste homolog 2 (EZH2), hepsin, and thymosin-beta 15.[11] Men searching prostate cancer websites for news of current research will see frequent references to these proteins.

Probably the most promising future technique for predicting prostate cancers is the use of gene and protein expression. With microarray techniques, thousands of genes and proteins are put onto a microchip. Tissue from a prostate cancer is then also put onto the chip, showing which specific genes or proteins are activated. The hope is that specific combinations of genes and proteins, commonly referred to as gene expression profiles, will be identified and will be useful in predicting the probable future course of any given cancer. In late 2004 this technology became available for predicting the recurrence of breast cancer, and it is likely to become available for prostate cancer in the near future.

Another approach to improving prediction has been to refine imaging techniques so that they can be used to assess the size of prostate cancers and predict their future course. To date, the use of traditional computerized tomography (CT) and magnetic resonance imaging (MRI) has been disappointing. Researchers have begun using nanoparticles called lymphotrophic superparamagnetic nanoparticles (LSNs), which enter into lymph cells and can be seen on MRI; whether this procedure can predict the spread of prostate cancer to lymph nodes is being investigated.

The variety of research offers much hope for the future. Men in their 50s or younger are almost certainly going to benefit and will have far more precise means to both diagnose and predict the course of their cancer. Those of us who are older may or may not benefit, but we have the satisfaction of knowing that our sons and grandsons will not experience the uncertainties that we have faced. This is no small progress.

The Anatomy and Function of the Prostate Gland

Michelangelo's *David* notwithstanding, the anatomy of the human male leaves a lot to be desired. Our organs of reproduction and recreation are hopelessly intertwined with our organs of liquid waste disposal. As one observer facetiously noted, "Only a Civil Engineer could have designed the body [since] who else would design a waste disposal line through a recreational area?"[1]

Sitting in the center of this anatomical assemblage is the prostate, a reddish-brown organ approximately an inch and a half in diameter. It lies at the bottom of the pelvis, with the penis below, the bladder above, the pelvic bone in front, and the rectum behind (Figure 3). This last juxtaposition is especially important, because feeling the prostate through the rectal wall—the much-maligned digital rectal exam—is the only way a physician can physically assess this organ. Fortunately, the majority of cancers develop in the posterior portion of the prostate, thereby making them detectable to a skilled examining finger.

The prostate has been variously described as looking like a walnut, a chestnut, or a small plum. In a young man, it weighs approximately 20 gm, then increases in size as the man ages. It contains muscles and glands, the latter secreting fluid that assists and protects male sperm. One component of the prostate fluid is prostate specific antigen (PSA), described in Chapter 2.

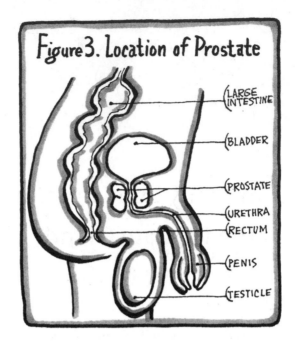

The prostate contributes approximately one third of the fluid that makes up the semen. The other two thirds comes from the paired seminal vesicles, small glands that sit at the base of the bladder and drain through the prostate into the urethra. Joining the seminal vesicle ducts in the prostate are the paired vasa deferentia, which carry sperm from the testicles. The vasa deferentia, seminal vesicle ducts, and ducts from the internal prostate glands all join together at the urethra in the middle of the prostate (Figure 4).

Thus, the prostate center is the Grand Central Station of the male reproductive system. There, at the time of orgasm, sperm and the accompanying fluid begin their journey down the urethra, through the penis, and with luck up the vagina and uterus, perhaps to find a waiting egg in the fallopian tubes. According to *Dr. Peter Scardino's Prostate Book,* the sperm travel "at the startling rate of 28 miles per hour, which, by amusing coincidence, is also the top speed a world-class human runner can achieve during a sprint."[2]

This complicated system would work fine, except for the fact that the urethra has a second function, as the exit for urine. Filtered by the kidneys and then deposited into the bladder, which sits on top

What a Curious Organ

I would like to sit down with my doctor and talk to him about the prostate. What a curious organ. What can God have been thinking when He designed it this way?

—Anatole Broyard, *Intoxicated by My Illness*

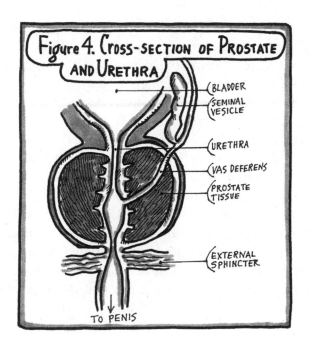

Figure 4. Cross-section of Prostate and Urethra

of the prostate, urine passes via the urethra directly through the middle of the prostate. To avoid a constant dribble of urine, the muscles at the base of the bladder function as an internal sphincter (although technically they are not a true sphincter). The urethra also has an external sphincter, a true sphincter, just below the prostate. Both sphincters must relax for urination to take place.

When one or both sphincters are damaged, as during surgical

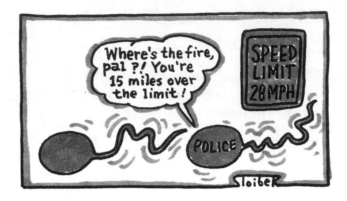

removal of the prostate, or are not working properly, which may happen as a side effect of medication, the result may be some degree of incontinence. During orgasm and ejaculation, the external sphincter opens to allow the semen to leave, while the internal sphincter closes to prevent semen from flowing upward into the bladder. When the sphincters do not work properly, semen may flow into the bladder; this is called retrograde ejaculation. It is harmless, but obviously does not result in the fertilization of female eggs. Alternatively, if the internal sphincter does not close during orgasm, urine may descend through the urethra, a common but usually temporary complication of surgical removal of the prostate (see Chapter 3).

But this anatomical anarchy actually is even worse. Running close to the sides of the prostate are tiny arteries, veins, and nerves that go to the penis and control erection. If they are damaged during surgical removal or irradiation of the prostate, the man may achieve only a partial erection or no erection at all. This impotence is a common side effect of prostate cancer treatment, as discussed in Chapter 10.

Given this anatomy, it becomes apparent why enlargement of the prostate, due to either benign prostatic hypertrophy (BPH) or cancer, may cause serious problems. An enlargement of the prostate may squeeze the urethra, thereby making the urinary stream progressively smaller and urination more difficult. This process occurs commonly in aging men, since the prostate begins to enlarge during middle age. The reason for this enlargement is unknown; it is caused by testosterone stimulation but appears to serve no useful evolutionary purpose other than to make urology a necessary medical specialty.

Given this anatomy, it also becomes apparent why treating prostate cancer can so often lead to incontinence and impotence. It is virtually impossible to surgically excise, irradiate, or otherwise remove a cancerous growth in the prostate without damaging surrounding structures. As one observer summarized the situation: "God's specialty was humanity, not urology."[3]

Most people assume that prostate cancer is a disease exclusively of men. This is not quite true. In the first few weeks of development in utero, males and females are exactly alike. The anatomy of both develops from the same structures. Therefore, there are remnants of female structures in males, and remnants of male structures in females. In women, the remnants of the prostate are tiny, paired paraurethral glands that lie beside the urethra. Rarely, these glands can become cancerous, the result being a female equivalent of prostate cancer. Approximately sixty such cases have been described in the medical literature. Thus, we have equality between the sexes: men can (rarely) get breast cancer, and women can (rarely) get the equivalent of prostate cancer.

Evaluation of Books
About Prostate Cancer

The following, listed alphabetically by author, are assessments of forty-seven books about prostate cancer published in the past seven years (asterisks indicate those I have found most valuable). Also included are a few volumes published earlier that are of special interest. Books on prostate health in general are not included.

Alterowitz, Ralph, and Alterowitz, Barbara. *The Lovin' Ain't Over: The Couples Guide to Better Sex After Prostate Disease.* Westbury, N.Y.: Health Education Literary Publisher, 1999. Written by a man who has had prostate cancer and his wife, this book focuses exclusively on impotence. It explains the complexities of erections and orgasms and outlines options for couples faced with varying degrees of impotence.

Baggish, Jeff. *Making the Prostate Therapy Decision* (rev. ed.). Los Angeles: Lowell House, 1998. Originally published in 1995, this book was said to have been revised in 1998. The changes, however, appear to have been minimal and the book is now outdated.

Barrett, David M. (ed.) *Mayo Clinic on Prostate Health.* Rochester, Minn.: Mayo Clinic, 2000. This slim (166-page) book is inadequate in most respects. Only half of it is about prostate cancer: a little bit about everything, not enough about anything. Its priorities are difficult to understand. For example, it allocates only four pages to radiation beam and seed therapy combined, but eight pages to complementary treatments. No references or notes are given.

Bodai, Ernie. *I Flunked my PSA!* Severna Park, Md.: B2Z Publishing, 2002. This thin volume was written by a surgeon who had prostate cancer. Although advertised as a "prostate cancer primer," it provides too little information on most subjects. Reading the book is rather like being served a small appetizer when you are hungry for the main course.

Bostwick, David G.; Crawford, E. David; Higano, Celestia S.; and Roach, Mark (eds.). *American Cancer Society's Complete Guide to Prostate Cancer.* Atlanta: American Cancer Society, 2005. This revised and updated edition of the American Cancer Society's 1996 book is solid as far as it goes. However, many men will want more detailed data. For instance, no five-, ten-, or fifteen-year survival rate figures appear; little mention is made of treatment studies that compare one type of treatment with another; and no numbered references allow one to follow up on any given fact or figure. Thus, the book lacks specific information to help a man choose which treatment is best for him. These shortcomings may be an inevitable consequence of having sixty-two authors and trying not to offend anyone.

*Broyard, Anatole. *Intoxicated by My Illness.* New York: Ballantine Books, 1992. This book is a little classic. The author was a book critic for the *New York Times* when, at age 69, he was diagnosed with advanced prostate cancer. He died fourteen months later, after having written the first four essays in this book. He yearned for "an untamed, beautiful death" and suggested that "we should have a competition in dying, sort of like Halloween costumes. . . . Let's give a prize for the most beautiful death. We can call it heaven."

Bubley, Glenn J., with Conkling, Winifred. *What Your Doctor May Not Tell You About Prostate Cancer: The Breakthrough Information and Treatments That Can Help Save Your Life.* New York: Warner Books, 2005. This book was written by a Boston oncologist whose practice includes many patients with recurrent prostate cancer. For such men it is a useful book, since it contains excellent chapters on experimental treatments and clinical trials. The chapters on natural remedies (herbs, vitamins, and minerals), dietary factors, and support groups are also recommended. The author summarizes traditional treatments in an unbiased but somewhat sketchy manner. The weakest element is the histrionic title—the book is, in fact, much better than its cover would suggest.

Centeno, Arthur, and Onik, Gary. *Prostate Cancer: A Patient's*

Guide to Treatment. Omaha: Addicus Books, 2004. Written by a urologist and a radiologist, both of whom specialize in prostate cancer, this book too offers a little of everything but not enough of anything. It tends to minimize the seriousness of side effects and complications of the various treatments. It is sympathetic to cryosurgery; Onik was one of the developers of this treatment.

Connell, Will. *Prostate Cancer Treatment Options: A Guide to the Basics.* Grass Valley, Calif.: Edconco Press, 1997. Written by an engineer who had prostate cancer, this book's strength is that it helps men rationally think through their treatment options and decide what is best for them. Its weakness is that it is somewhat out of date.

Dattoli, Michael; Cash, Jennifer; and Kaltenbach, Don. *Surviving Prostate Cancer Without Surgery.* Sarasota, Fla.: Seneca Press, 2005. This book is a companion to *Prostate Cancer: A Survivor's Guide,* by Kaltenbach and Richards. Both are publications of Dattoli's cancer treatment center, which specializes in radiation seed therapy combined with beam radiation. As such, the authors extol the merits of brachytherapy ("Side effects with [seed] implants are usually mild and reversible") and denigrate surgical treatment.

*Dorso, Michael A. *Seeds of Hope: A Physician's Personal Triumph over Prostate Cancer.* Battle Creek, Mich.: Acorn Publishing, 2000. This book was written by an emergency room physician who, at age 54, had a Gleason 6 prostate cancer and elected to use a combination of hormones, beam radiation, and radiation seed therapy. He writes honestly and well about his decision-making steps, the advantages and disadvantages of his approach, and the effects of the cancer on his wife and himself. It is an especially useful book for men considering radiation seed therapy.

Ellsworth, Pamela; Heaney, John; and Gill, Cliff. *100 Questions and Answers About Prostate Cancer.* Sudbury, Mass.: Jones and Bartlett, 2003. Written by two urologists and a man who chose surgery for his prostate cancer, this book includes useful information but is oddly organized. The question-and-answer format makes it difficult to find the information you want and leads to a great deal of repetition. Much of the information is presented in charts that I personally found sterile and unsatisfying.

Fisher, William L. *How To Fight Prostate Cancer and Win.* Baltimore: Agora Books, 2001. This book is mistitled and includes relatively little about prostate cancer. It covers benign prostatic hypertrophy and prostate health in general, emphasizing herbal and dietary approaches.

*Gottlicb, Bert, and Mawn, Thomas J. *The Men's Club: How To Lose Your Prostate Without Losing Your Sense of Humor.* Oxnard, Calif.: Pathfinder Publishing, 1999. This is an entertaining account of a radical prostatectomy followed by ongoing incontinence and implantation of an artificial sphincter. Injecting humor into such a sequence is a major challenge, but the authors succeed. Gottlieb was a 61-year-old advertising executive when diagnosed with a Gleason 5 cancer, and alternate sections are written by Mawn, his urologist. Patient and physician developed a close and mutually affectionate relationship. Gottlieb's wife plays a significant role in getting her husband through the ordeal with both love and levity. She even gets Mawn to promise that he will have no more than one glass of wine the night before the surgery.

Gray, Ross. *Prostate Tales: Men's Experiences with Prostate Cancer.* Harriman, Tenn.: Men's Studies Press, 2003. This collection of short stories about men with prostate cancer is similar to those to be found on many prostate cancer websites. These, however, have been edited by the author, a researcher in Toronto, and are much more readable. The author says that he "wanted to make the struggles and triumphs of men with prostate cancer more visible to men themselves and more understandable to others"; he has succeeded in doing so.

Grimm, Peter D.; Blasko, John C.; and Sylvester, John E. (eds). *The Prostate Cancer Treatment Book.* New York: McGraw Hill, 2004. As an up-to-date guide to treatment options, this book is useful. It focuses especially on radiation seed therapy and work at the Seattle Prostate Institute, the home of the editors. As such, it has a cheerleader tone, with an implication that everything important is done at their headquarters. Each chapter is multiauthored by a different group, so the writing styles vary considerably. The book includes no information about causes, focusing exclusively on treatments.

Handy, Richard Y. *Prostate Cancer: Treatment and Recovery.* Amherst, N.Y.: Prometheus Books, 1996 (originally published in 1988). Diagnosed with prostate cancer at age 52, the author had a prostatectomy followed by radiation that left him permanently impotent. His account focuses on the effects of the impotence on his wife and himself, and he recounts with ruthless honesty the indignities, depressions, and vulnerabilities that followed. His preoccupation with his penis is a Freudian's delight, and men who suffer impotence as a consequence of their cancer will find the book useful.

Hennefent, Bradley. *Surviving Prostate Cancer Without Surgery.* Roseville, Ill.: Roseville Books, 2005. This is an odd book in that its main message is a diatribe against surgical treatment. For example: "Consider the magnified humiliation of radical prostatectomy patients. Not only has their money been taken, but their penises have been crippled and their sex lives have been largely destroyed." The author, an emergency room physician, was inspired to write the book by his uncle, who "died from his prostate cancer treatment."

*Hersh, Stephen P. *Beyond Miracles: Living with Cancer.* Santa Ana, Calif.: Seven Locks Press, 2000. Of the many books aimed at survivors of cancer in general, not just prostate cancer, this is among the best. Written by a psychiatrist and specialist in cancer patients and pain management, it encourages patients to take an active role both in managing their cancer treatment plan and in managing stress.

Hitchcock, Robert. *Love, Sex, and PSA.* San Diego: TMC Press, 1997. This is a brief, light book written by a 61-year-old playwright who got prostate cancer (Gleason 5, PSA 7.7). It includes a straight-talking and sometimes humorous section on impotence and its possible treatments (the author used self-injections successfully).

Horowitz, David. *The End of Time.* San Francisco: Encounter Books, 2005. Horowitz was 62 years old when he was diagnosed with prostate cancer (Gleason 7, PSA 6.0) and had a radical prostatectomy and post-op radiation. This book covers very little about his cancer but rather is a series of meditations on life, death, and love. It is nicely written but of limited value to men looking for information.

Howe, Desiree Lyon, *His Prostate and Me.* Houston: Winedale Publishing, 2002. Written in a chatty style by the wife of a man with prostate cancer, the book, as the title suggests, is aimed at wives. It starts slowly, but the second half includes an extensive and useful account of how Howe coped with her husband's postsurgical incontinence and impotence. For women confronted with these situations, the book will be helpful.

Kaltenbach, Don, with Richards, Tom. *Prostate Cancer: A Survivor's Guide.* Sarasota, Fla.: Seneca House Press, 2003 (originally published in 1996). The author, who wrote this book with the help of a professional writer, was a lawyer who was diagnosed with prostate cancer in his early 40s. He chose radiation seed therapy, and the book is strongly biased toward this treatment. Kaltenbach, in fact, now works for a surgical group specializing in this treatment, so the text has some of the flavor of an advertisement. The most useful part is a section on costs and insurance coverage of prostate cancer treatment.

Klein, Eric A.; Jamnicky, Leah; and Nam, Robert. *So You're Having Prostate Surgery.* Hoboken, N.J.: John Wiley, 2003. Written by two urologists and a urology nurse, this slim volume is targeted at men who have elected to have surgery. Thus, it is surprising that a third of the book covers other issues. It has a folksy style ("We know—you're tough and can handle a lot"). The pages are printed in green on white, which may appeal if you are Irish. Overall, moderately helpful but not essential reading.

*Korda, Michael. *Man to Man: Surviving Prostate Cancer.* New York: Vintage Books, 1996. This is a widely read account of the author's radical prostatectomy. He was a 61-year-old publishing executive with prostate cancer (Gleason 6, PSA 22), for which he elected surgery. The author is brutally honest in detailing his problems and reactions, and when the book was originally published, it was one of the first such books available. Korda had major post-op problems with incontinence and thus makes prostatectomy sound worse than many other men have reported. Still, the text contains much that is helpful.

*Lange, Paul H., and Adamec, Christine. *Prostate Cancer for Dummies.* New York: John Wiley, 2003. Written by a well-known urologist who himself had prostate cancer and a medical writer whose husband had prostate cancer, this is one of the most widely read books. It is user friendly, with a detailed (ten-page) table of contents, lots of boxes, and icons indicating technical material that can be skipped.

Lewis, James. *The Herbal Remedy for Prostate Cancer.* Westbury, N.Y.: Health Education Literary Publisher, 1999. This book is essentially a 200-page advertisement for PC-SPES, an herbal remedy promoted for use in prostate cancer. Since PC-SPES was subsequently taken off the market by the Food and Drug Administration because it had been adulterated with dangerous medications, the information in this book is now moot.

Lintzenich, Joseph W. *Oh No, Not Me.* San Jose, Calif.: Writers

Club Press, 2001. The author was a 55-year-old pilot in 1992 when he was diagnosed with prostate cancer and subsequently had surgery. This is his account—pleasant and chatty, but somewhat long-winded. Readers are not really interested in how the author names his dogs or this level of detail: "John blew the horn at 2:35 and Pat handed me my coat and I was out the door." In its favor, the author provides the most detailed account available of his days immediately after surgery. He deals frankly with his incontinence and impotence, both of which were resolved; as such, the book is a counterpoint to Korda's *Man to Man.*

Loo, Marcus H., and Betancourt, Marian. *The Prostate Cancer Source Book.* New York: John Wiley, 1998. This is a practical and well-written summary of treatment options for prostate cancer, emphasizing surgery. It is especially worthwhile on little details that most books overlook, such as recommending that you bring a CD player to the hospital for your stay and, if possible, schedule your surgery as the first case in the morning so that you won't have to wait. Unfortunately, the work is now out of date on many treatment issues.

*Marks, Sheldon. *Prostate and Cancer: A Family Guide to Diagnosis, Treatment, and Survival* (3rd ed.). New York: Perseus, 2003. Originally published in 1995, this is one of the best books available on prostate cancer. It is user friendly, with forty chapters in question-and-answer format and a helpful index. Like most books written by urologists, it primarily covers treatment issues and includes little on causes (except nutrition), research, and other issues.

Martin, William. *My Prostate and Me.* New York: Cadell and Davies, 1994. This account of prostate cancer was written by a sociology professor in his 40s. With a Gleason score of 7 and a PSA of 8, he elected to have a radical prostatectomy. His account is useful but rather long-winded and would have benefited from a firm editor.

McClure, Mark W. *Smart Medicine for a Healthy Prostate.* New York: Avery Penguin Putnam, 2001. Written by a urologist who supports complementary and holistic medicine, only one third of this book is about prostate cancer. It covers in detail diet, vitamins, herbs, and lifestyle changes that some men have found helpful.

Neider, Charles. *Adam's Burden: An Explorer's Personal Odyssey Through Prostate Cancer.* Lanham, Md.: Madison Books, 2001. The author, an adventurer and writer, was diagnosed with prostate cancer (Gleason 6, PSA 16) at age 78 and died from it at age 86. The diary account of his beam radiation treatment may be useful for men considering this treatment. The book could have used a thorough editing, as most readers may not be interested in what the weather was each day, what the author was reading, and the like.

Newton, Audrey Currie. *Living with Prostate Cancer*. Toronto: McClelland and Stewart, 1996. Written by his wife, this book tells of a Canadian man who at age 59 was diagnosed with prostate cancer that had spread to his lymph nodes. With radiation treatments and hormone suppression, he lived ten more years. Two years after being diagnosed with prostate cancer, he was diagnosed with bowel cancer. His personal story is interspersed with chapters of factual material, now outdated, about prostate cancer.

Nixon, Daniel W., and Gomez, Max. *The Prostate Health Program: A Guide to Preventing and Controlling Prostate Cancer*. New York: Free Press, 2004. This book was written by a physician who is president of the Institute of Cancer Prevention and by a science reporter. As one might surmise, the majority of the book focuses on healthy diets and lifestyles. It has a worthwhile chapter on alternative treatments for prostate cancer but is comparatively weak on standard treatments and their complications.

Osterling, Joseph E., and Moyad, Mark A. *The ABCs of Prostate Cancer: The Book That Could Save Your Life*. Lanham, Md.: Madison Books, 1997. Written by a urologist whose father died of prostate cancer and a public health educator, this widely read book is now out-of-date. It has many strengths, including testimonials by famous and not-so-famous people who have had prostate cancer. However, it is cumbersome and somewhat repetitious—and a pharmaceutical company logo on the back raises questions about objectivity.

Perlman, Gerald, and Drescher, Jack (eds.). *A Gay Man's Guide to Prostate Cancer*. Binghamton, N.Y.: Haworth Press, 2005. This book is essential reading for gay men who are diagnosed with prostate cancer. The series of stories written by gay men of varying ages and professions includes a social worker, psychologist, psychiatrist, economist, and urologist. All of them frankly discuss gay concerns that bear on their diagnosis, including concurrent AIDS and their sexuality. Many of the authors have also been involved in Malecare, Inc., a nonprofit support group (see www.malecare.com).

Pienta, Kenneth J., and Moyad, Mark A. *Prostate Cancer from A to Z*. Ann Arbor, Mich.: Media Group, 2004. This uneven book provides reasonably full information on some subjects (PSA interpretation, hormone treatment) but bare bones on other subjects (surgery, radiation treatment). It oversimplifies survival statistics and includes no references for men who want to delve in more detail. The book also provides no perspective on the relative importance of many subjects. For example, shark cartilage, with no evidence that it is useful in prostate cancer, is listed alongside lycopene, for which evidence of its utility does exist.

Pilgrim, Aubrey. *A Revolutionary Approach to Prostate Cancer*. Pittsburgh: SterlingHouse, 1997. Written by a chiropractor who had prostate cancer, this book has a chatty style but is somewhat disorganized. The type is very small and there are few visuals. Like most prostate books, it focuses almost exclusively on diagnosis and treatment. Its special strengths are an interesting chapter on "quackery" and a lengthy list of resources.

Prochnik, Leon. *You Can't Make Love if You're Dead*. Los Angeles: Ari Press, 2000. Written by a Hollywood screenplay writer with prostate cancer (Gleason 6, PSA 11), this brief book recounts his search for the right treatment. Predictably, each doctor he consulted suggested a different course. His ultimate advice came from his aunt, who recommended surgery, her reasoning later being used as the title of the book.

Ryan, Cornelius, and Ryan, Kathryn Morgan. *A Private Battle*. New York: Simon and Schuster, 1979. Cornelius Ryan was a successful writer when, at age 50, he was diagnosed with advanced prostate cancer. The result is this book written by Ryan and his wife, also a writer, about the subsequent four years until he died. The events took place from 1970 to 1974, and what is striking is how different, and yet how much the same, everything is. We forget the far greater stigma surrounding cancer thirty-five years ago; the Ryans initially kept the diagnosis a secret from even their closest friends. On the other hand, each urologist Ryan consulted urged a different course of treatment, similar to the situation many men encounter today. During his battle with cancer, Ryan wrote *A Bridge Too Far,* which, at the time of his death, was second on the nationwide best-seller list. Ryan's editor for that book was Michael Korda, who, two decades later, would write a book about his own prostate cancer.

*Scardino, Peter T., and Kelman, Judith. *Dr. Peter Scardino's Prostate Book: The Complete Guide to Overcoming Prostate Cancer, Prostatitis, and BPH*. New York: Avery, 2005. With the retirement of Patrick Walsh as the de facto dean of American prostate cancer, Peter Scardino appears to be applying to assume that role. The similar book titles, the cowriting of both books with professional writers, and many allusions to the treatment superiority of Scardino's Memorial Sloan-Kettering Cancer Center in New York over Walsh's Johns Hopkins Medical Center in Baltimore and other centers all suggest a usurper to the prostate cancer throne. What the two books share is a strong bias toward surgery as the best treatment for most men. That being said, there is much valuable information in the Scardino book plus a useful glossary and index, and the information is up-to-date as of late 2004. The shortcomings include weak sections on causes, hormone treatment, and resources, and few personal stories. Although well written, there is much duplication of information, which contributes to its almost five-hundred-page bulk—yet another feature it shares with the Walsh and Worthington book.

Strum, Stephen B., and Pogliano, Donna. *A Primer on Prostate Cancer: The Empowered Patient's Guide*. Hollywood, Fla.: Life Extension Foundation, 2002. This visually appealing book has pictures, diagrams, and even some multicolor text. Strum is an oncologist and a pioneer in hormone therapy. The book is almost exclusively devoted to diagnosis and treatment and in parts is quite technical. Publication was partially funded by the Prostate Cancer Research Institute, cofounded by the senior author, and the book appears to be biased toward radiation and hormone therapy.

Wainrib, Barbara, and Haber, Sandra. *Men, Women, and Prostate Cancer*. Oakland, Calif.: New Harbinger, 2000. This is a modestly updated edition of a 1996 book, *Prostate Cancer: A Guide for Women and the Men They Love*. It is written by two female psychologists who previously published a book on breast cancer. Aimed at the wives of men affected with prostate cancer, it is especially heavy on emotional issues and staying psychologically healthy. The best chapter has suggestions for responding to a man's impotence.

*Walsh, Patrick C., and Worthington, Janet F. *Dr. Patrick Walsh's Guide to Surviving Prostate Cancer*. New York: Time Warner, 2001. This is one of the most widely read books on prostate cancer. Although it has many strong points, it is wordy, redundant, and weighty (443 pages). Worthington is a science writer at Johns Hopkins Medical Center, and Walsh is the former chief of urology there. The book strongly reflects the surgical interests of the senior author and in some sections has the tone of a cheerleader. It includes much valuable information but has some omissions (such as the possible role of sexually transmitted diseases) and strong biases (it is overly enthusiastic about dietary causes). It is also unduly sanguine about outcomes and postoperative complications following prostatectomy.

*Wheeler, Chuck, and Wheeler, Martha. *Affirming the Darkness: An Extended Conversation About Living with Prostate Cancer.* Beverly, Mass.: Memoirs Unlimited, 1996. This is a book in which the husband and wife, married for fifty years, kept separate diaries. Chuck Wheeler was diagnosed with a Gleason 9 prostate cancer at age 65 and died eight years later. This account of those years includes his surgery, penile prosthesis, orchiectomy, metastasis, and pain control. At one point Chuck writes: "You know, honey, I've never died before. This is a brand-new experience for me. It's a constant preoccupation." This excellent book about dying from prostate cancer should be read by anyone who doubts that the disease can be nasty and deadly.

Williams, Charles R., and Williams, Vernon A. *That Black Men Might Live.* Roscoe, Ill.: Hilton Publishing, 2003. Rev. Charles Williams has written a cautionary tale aimed at black men but applicable to all men. He initially ignored multiple signs and symptoms that something was seriously wrong with his urinary tract. When he finally had a PSA taken, it was 172. What did he do next? He ignored it for five additional months. When at last he had a biopsy, the prostate cancer had already spread to his bones. Trying to salvage something from this personal disaster, Rev. Williams dedicated the remainder of his life to educating other black men about the importance of regular PSA testing. The writing is uneven, but the message comes through loud and clear.

Useful Websites on Prostate Cancer

Like many men of my era, I am Internet challenged and relatively website illiterate. I do not understand, for example, why you click Start on the computer when what you want to do is Stop. The following evaluation of websites on prostate cancer is therefore based on my amateur status; accomplished Internet experts may disagree with my conclusions.

Literally dozens of websites provide information on prostate cancer. Like all websites, they come and go, so do not be surprised if you are unable to find some of those mentioned here.

There is much useful information on the Internet; there is also much misinformation. One of the biggest challenges in evaluating websites is to ascertain who sponsors them. Many of the prostate cancer websites are sponsored by specific treatment centers, types of treatment, or pharmaceutical companies. These sites therefore have commercial interests, although sometimes not obviously. Valuable information may be presented but, by definition, you are not being given a balanced point of view because the website has something to sell. The following assessments thus include only those websites that do not appear to be unduly influenced by commercial interests. The only exceptions are sites that include unique information not available elsewhere, such as www.centerwatch.com (information on drug trials) and www.fightprostatecancer.org (advocacy).

Specifically *excluded* are the following:

- Websites that advocate a specific treatment, for example, www.cryocarepca.org, which promotes cryosurgery, or www.ecpcp.org, which promotes alternative therapies.
- Websites that tout specific treatment centers; examples are www.oncolink.upenn.edu, which promotes the cancer treatment center at the University of Pennsylvania, and www.prci.org (also accessed by www.prostate-cancer.org), which promotes the Prostate Cancer Research Institute in Los Angeles.
- Websites that promote specific drugs, devices, and/or publications, and where commercial interests would be expected to influence the information they provide, for instance, www.prostateforum.com, www.cancerfacts.com, and www.seekwellness.com.

Many prostate cancer websites include electronic newsletters, mailing lists, message boards, blogs, listservs, chat rooms, and on-line discussion groups. These can be very helpful, especially for men who are geographically isolated from support groups and comprehensive libraries. But again, beware of commercial interests; if a website is trying to sell you something, you have clicked your way into a business and not a classroom. Many of the most valuable websites accept donations. Helping them out is an effective way to keep them independent.

The following, then, are the most useful websites on prostate cancer among the more than forty sites I examined. Those marked with an asterisk (at the beginning of the list) are those that appeared to me to be the best.

*www.cancer.gov (also accessed through www.nih.nci.gov)
This is the site of the National Cancer Institute, a component of the National Institutes of Health. Well designed, it allows you to immediately select the type of cancer on which you want information. The sections on treatment under "Cancer Topics" are excellent and provide a simple "Patient Version," a more detailed "Health Professional Version," and an "En Español" version. The section on "Clinical Trials" allows you to specify your type of cancer and the stage. When you input your zip code, the site gives you all the trials within a given

number of miles (which you specify) of that zip code. The section "Treatment Facilities" provides the names and addresses of the official cancer centers, designated by the National Cancer Institute, as explained in Chapter 8. Another section on "Cancer Statistics" gives you more than you ever wanted to know. Overall, this website is the best for reliable information on prostate cancer.

*www.cancer.prostate-help.org (formerly www.prostate-help.org)
This private site was created by Don Cooley of San Jose, California, after he was diagnosed with prostate cancer in 1997. He advertises it as "the largest noncommercial, individually owned and operated" site, and it is indeed huge. It is well organized and easy to navigate with gateways (such as "Patients Helping Patients") that lead to specific topics ("Surgical Removal of the Prostate") that in turn lead to subtopics ("Who Should/Should Not Have Surgery"). In early 2006 the gateways were under revision to make it even easier to find what you want. The site includes groups and chat rooms. Cooley prides himself on including only proven scientific data on his site and does not shy away from controversies. Overall, this website is a labor of love on which Cooley claims to have spent "over 6 years of 10- to 16-hour days." He accepts donations, but these are not tax deductible because he does not have tax-exempt status.

*www.phoenix5.org
This private website was created in 2000 by Robert Young after he was diagnosed with prostate cancer (with a PSA of over 1,000). It is exceptionally practical, with, for example, a listing of prostate cancer support groups by state and evaluations of other websites. Its principal assets are personal stories written by prostate cancer survivors and their wives/partners, but it also includes links to news stories on prostate cancer. The site is especially strong on the effects of prostate cancer on masculinity and sexual function.

*www.ustoo.org
This is the best site for locating a prostate cancer support group. It is maintained by Us Too International Inc. in Downers Grove, Illinois, which advertises itself as the "oldest and largest cancer education and support network." It claims 330 support groups, which can be

identified by clicking on individual states. The site is less useful than some others for obtaining objective treatment information, because it is linked with websites that have commercial interests.

www.cancer.org

This website of the American Cancer Society is not well designed but, with patience, yields much useful information. Its strongest feature is "Medical Updates," which includes summaries of important prostate cancer news stories of the past few years. When I accessed it in 2005, however, this feature appeared to be relatively deficient in recent stories. The website includes message boards and, if you look hard enough, the location of the American Cancer Society–sponsored Man to Man support groups. Finding a group in my area required a great deal of trial-and-error hunting; I finally located one under the heading "In My Community."

www.cpcn.org

This is the website of the Canadian Prostate Cancer Network (CPCN), which is the national association of prostate cancer support groups. For Canadians who are looking for a support group, here is the place to begin.

www.hypertext.org

This site was organized in 1997 by Bill Dyckes, who was diagnosed with prostate cancer and elected to have radioactive seed implants. In acknowledgments for the site, Dykes thanks his urologist "who, by seeming to have so little interest in my illness, forced me to learn about it for myself." Information on the site is in Spanish and Portuguese as well as English. Basic information is available, with links to many other sites for more detailed information. A nice feature is a pull-down menu that allows the user to select specific topics. However, when I accessed the site in 2005, some topics had not been updated in more than two years.

www.nccn.org

This is the site of the National Comprehensive Cancer Network, an organization of nineteen leading cancer treatment centers in the United States. The most useful aspect of the site is "Treatment Guidelines for Patients" by cancer type, which is available on-line and can be requested by mail as a booklet. The site is maintained by dues from the nineteen cancer centers, so its views reflect mainstream cancer treatment. You can also access the ongoing treatment trials at each of the centers; all should also be listed on the much more inclusive www.cancer.gov section on "Clinical Trials."

www.centerwatch.com
This commercial website, "a business of The Thomson Corporation," is included because it lists existing clinical drug trials, including those sponsored by pharmaceutical companies and not the National Cancer Institute. To access those for prostate cancer, click first on "Oncology" and then on "Prostate Cancer." The treatment trials are listed by state.

www.paactusa.org
Founded in 1983 by Lloyd Ney when he was diagnosed with late-stage prostate cancer, this website promotes treatments for similar late-stage cases. Most of the information is through links. Ney died in 1998, and it is unclear whether this website is being appropriately updated.

www.yananow.net
This site was set up by Australian Gregg Morrison and his wife. He was diagnosed with prostate cancer at age 61 and opted for surgery. Having had complications and recurrences, he says that in retrospect he wishes he had chosen another form of treatment. The website contains some useful information but is not as complete as many others.

www.fightprostatecancer.org (www.pcacoalition.org)
The National Prostate Cancer Coalition (NPCC) was founded in 1996 to focus on education, public awareness, and political advocacy to promote research on prostate cancer. Its website includes links to many other helpful sites such as Phoenix 5 and Public Citizen. It was completely updated and redesigned in 2005. You can sign up to receive NPCC's weekly on-line newsletter "Aware," the finest prostate cancer newsletter I have seen. This website is the best one for individuals interested in education and advocacy efforts.

www.prostatecancerfoundation.org (formerly www.capcure.org)
This is the site of the Prostate Cancer Foundation, begun by Michael
Milken in 1993 after he was diagnosed with advanced prostate cancer (see Chapter 14). It is useful primarily for individuals interested in
promoting research on prostate cancer and especially in finding new
drugs to control and/or cure it. The foundation accepts donations.

www.citizen.org
This is the website of Public Citizen Health Research Group. It includes useful information on the side effects of medications ("Good
Pills, Bad Pills"), dietary and herbal supplements, and a comparison
of the actions of state medical boards in disciplining doctors.

NOTES

1. On Being Diagnosed

1. David Horowitz, *The End of Time* (San Francisco: Encounter Books, 2005), 52.

2. Peter T. Scardino and Judith Kelman, *Dr. Peter Scardino's Prostate Book* (New York: Avery, 2005), 174; R. K. Nam, M. A. Jewett, M. D. Krahn, et al., Delay in surgical therapy for clinically localized prostate cancer and bio-chemical recurrence after radical prostatectomy, *Canadian Journal of Urology* 10 (2003): 1891–98; M. Graefen, J. Walz, K.-II. F. Chun, et al., Reasonable delay of surgical treatment in men with localized prostate cancer—impact on prognosis? *European Urology* 47 (2005): 756–760; S. A. Boorjian, F. J. Bianco Jr., P. T. Scardino, et al., Does the time from biopsy to surgery affect bio-chemical recurrence after radical prostatectomy? *British Journal of Urology* 96 (2005): 773–776.

3. Leon Jaroff, The man's cancer, *Time*, April 1, 1996, http://www.usrf.org/news/010815-Norman_Schwarzkopf_CaP.html, accessed September 19, 2005.

4. Jan Hoffman, Awash in information, patients face a lonely, uncertain road, *New York Times*, August 14, 2005.

2. How Serious Is Your Cancer?

1. I. M. Thompson, D. K. Pauler, P. J. Goodman, et al., Prevalence of prostate cancer among men with a prostate-specific antigen level ≤4.0 ng per milliliter, *New England Journal of Medicine* 350 (2004): 2239–46; Joseph E. Osterling and Mark A. Moyad, *The ABCs of Prostate Cancer: The Book That Could Save Your Life* (Lanham, Md.: Madison Books, 1997), 2; A. J. Birtle, A. Freeman, J. R. W. Masters, et al., Clinical features of patients who present with metastatic prostate carcinoma and serum prostate-specific antigen (PSA) levels <10 ng/mL, *Cancer* 98 (2003): 2362–67.

2. M. K. Brawer, Prostate-specific antigen: current status, *CA—A Cancer Journal for Clinicians* 49 (1999): 264–281; Michael A. Dorso, *Seeds of Hope: A Physician's Personal Triumph over Prostate Cancer* (Battle Creek, Mich.: Acorn Publishing, 2000), 30.

3. H. B. Carter, J. D. Pearson, J. Metter, et al., Longitudinal evaluation of prostate-specific antigen levels in men with and without prostate diseases, *Journal of the American Medical Association* 267 (1992): 2215–20.

4. A. V. D'Amico, M.-H. Chen, K. A. Roehl, et al., Preoperative PSA velocity and the risk of death from prostate cancer after radical prostatectomy, *New England Journal of Medicine* 351 (2004): 125–135; A. V. D'Amico, A. A. Renshaw, B. Sussman, et al., Pretreatment PSA velocity and risk of death from prostate cancer following external beam radiation therapy, *Journal of the American Medical Association* 294 (2005): 440–447.

5. C. G. Ramos, K. A. Roehl, J. A. V. Antenor, et al., Percent carcinoma in prostatectomy specimen is associated with risk of recurrence after radical prostatectomy in patients with pathologically organ confined prostate cancer, *Journal of Urology* 172 (2004): 137–140; L. E. Eichelberger, M. O. Koch, J. K. Daggy, et al., Predicting tumor volume in radical prostatectomy specimens from patients with prostate cancer, *American Journal of Clinical Pathology* 120 (2003): 386–391; T. A. Stamey, J. E. McNeal, Cheryl M. Yemoto, et al., Biological determinants of cancer progression in men with prostate cancer, *Journal of the American Medical Association* 281 (1999): 1395–1400.

6. T. Y. Chan, A. W. Partin, P. C. Walsh, et al., Prognostic significance of Gleason score 3+4 versus Gleason score 4+3 tumor at radical prostatectomy, *Urology* 56 (2000): 823–827; L. Cheng, M. O. Koch, B. E. Juliar, et al., The combined percentage of Gleason patterns 4 and 5 is the best predictor of cancer progression after radical prostatectomy, *Journal of Clinical Oncology* 23 (2005): 2911–17.

7. M. Han, A. W. Partin, M. Zahurak, et al., Biochemical (prostate specific antigen) recurrence probability following radical prostatectomy for clinically localized prostate cancer, *Journal of Urology* 169 (2003): 517–523.

8. E. D. Grober, J. Tsihlias, M. A. S. Jewett, et al., Correlation of the primary Gleason pattern on prostate needle biopsy with clinico-pathological factors in Gleason 7 tumors, *Canadian Journal of Urology* 11 (2004): 2157–62; P. D. Sved, P. Gomez, M. Manoharan, et al., Limitations of biopsy Gleason grade: Implications for counseling patients with biopsy Gleason score 6 prostate cancer, *Journal of Urology* 172 (2004): 98–102; P. Sooriakumaran, D. P. Lovell, A. Henderson, et al., Gleason scoring varies among pathologists and this affects clinical risk in patients with prostate cancer, *Clinical Oncology* 17 (2005): 655–658.

9. Y. Lotan, S. F. Shariat, S. M. Khoddami, et al., The percent of biopsy cores positive for cancer is a predictor of advanced pathological stage and poor clinical outcomes in patients treated with radical prostatectomy, *Journal of Urology* 171 (2004): 2209–14; I. F. San Francisco, M. M. Regan, A. F. Olumi, et al., Percent of cores positive for cancer is a better preoperative predictor of cancer recurrence after radical prostatectomy than prostate specific antigen, *Journal of Urology* 171 (2004): 1492–99; S. J. Freedland, W. J. Aronson, M. K. Terris, et al., The percentage of prostate needle biopsy cores

with carcinoma from the more involved side of the biopsy as a predictor of prostate specific antigen recurrence after radical prostatectomy, *Cancer* 98 (2003): 2344–50; M. B. Gretzer, J. I. Epstein, C. R. Pound, et al., Substratification of Stage T1c prostate cancer based on the probability of biochemical recurrence, *Urology* 60 (2002): 1034–39; A. V. D'Amico, R. Whittington, S. B. Malkowicz, et al., Clinical utility of the percentage of positive prostate biopsies in defining biochemical outcome after radical prostatectomy for patients with clinically localized prostate cancer, *Journal of Clinical Oncology* 18 (2000): 1164–72; A. V. D'Amico, A. A. Renshaw, K. Cote, et al., Impact of the percentage of positive prostate cores on prostate cancer-specific mortality for patients with low or favorable intermediate-risk disease, *Journal of Clinical Oncology* 22 (2004): 3726–32.

10. J. W. Anast, G. L. Andriole, T. A. Bismar, et al., Relating biopsy and clinical variables to radical prostatectomy findings: Can insignificant and advanced prostate cancer be predicted in a screening population? *Urology* 64 (2004): 544–550; Gretzer et al., Substratification of Stage T1c prostate cancer.

3. Surgical Treatment

1. S. J. Freedland, J. C. Presti Jr., C. J. Kane, et al., Do younger men have better biochemical outcomes after radical prostatectomy? *Urology* 63 (2004): 518–522.

2. S. M. H. Alibhai, M. D. Krahn, M. M. Cohen, et al., Is there age bias in the treatment of localized prostate carcinoma? *Cancer* 100 (2004): 72–81.

3. M. Froehner, R. Koch, R. Litz, et al., Which conditions contributing to the Charlson score predict survival after radical prostatectomy? *Journal of Urology* 171 (2004): 697–699; Alibhai et al., Is there age bias?; Aubrey Pilgrim, *A Revolutionary Approach to Prostate Cancer* (Pittsburgh: SterlingHouse, 1997), 103.

4. A. M. Omar and N. Townell, Laparoscopic radical prostatectomy: A review of the literature and comparison with open techniques, *Prostate Cancer and Prostatic Diseases* 7 (2004): 295–301; R. Langreth, Men, cancer, and hope, *Forbes,* November 1, 2004.

5. Leon Jaroff, The man's cancer, *Time,* April 1, 1996, http://www.usrf .org/news/010815-Norman_Schwarzkopf_CaP.html, accessed September 19, 2005.

6. Bert Gottlieb and Thomas J. Mawn, *The Men's Club: How To Lose Your Prostate Without Losing Your Sense of Humor* (Oxnard, Calif.: Pathfinder, 1999), 102.

7. Patrick C. Walsh and Janet F. Worthington, *Dr. Patrick Walsh's Guide to Surviving Prostate Cancer* (New York: Time Warner, 2001), 226.

8. M. Savoie, S. S. Kim, M. S. Soloway, A prospective study measuring penile length in men treated with radical prostatectomy for prostate cancer, *Journal of Urology* 169 (2003): 1462–64; M. D. Munding, H. B. Wessells, B. L.

Dalkin, Pilot study of changes in stretched penile length 3 months after radical retropubic prostatectomy, *Urology* 58 (2001): 567–569; William Martin, *My Prostate and Me* (New York: Cadell and Davies, 1994), 186; N. Mondaini and P. Gontero, Re: A prospective study measuring penile length in men treated with radical prostatectomy for prostate cancer (letter), *Journal of Urology* 171 (2004): 359–360.

9. Martin, *My Prostate and Me,* 192.

10. Gottlieb and Mawn, *The Men's Club,* 125.

11. S. M. H. Alibhai, M. Leach, G. Tomlinson, et al., 30-day mortality and major complications after radical prostatectomy: Influence of age and comorbidity, *Journal of the National Cancer Institute* 97 (2005): 1525–32.

12. J. A. Talcott, P. Rieker, J. A. Clark, et al., Patient-reported symptoms after primary therapy for early prostate cancer: Results of a prospective cohort study, *Journal of Clinical Oncology* 16 (1998): 275–283.

13. P. C. Walsh, P. Marschke, D. Ricker, et al., Patient-reported urinary continence and sexual function after anatomic radical prostatectomy, *Urology* 55 (2000): 58–61; J. L. Stanford, Z. Feng, A. S. Hamilton, et al., Urinary and sexual function after radical prostatectomy for clinically localized prostate cancer: The Prostate Cancer Outcomes Study, *Journal of the American Medical Association* 283 (2000): 354–360; F. J. Fowler, M. J. Barry, G. Lu-Yao, et al., Patient-reported complications and follow-up treatment after radical prostatectomy: The National Medicare Experience: 1988–1990, *Urology* 42 (1993): 622–629; Talcott et al., Patient-reported symptoms; T. C. Kao, D. F. Cruess, D. Garner, et al., Multicenter patient self-reporting questionnaire on impotence, incontinence and stricture after radical prostatectomy, *Journal of Urology* 163 (2000): 858–864; J. C. Hu, E. P. Elkin, D. J. Pasta, Predicting quality of life after radical prostatectomy: Results from CaPSURE, *Journal of Urology* 171 (2004): 703–708.

14. B. K. Hollenbeck, R. L. Dunn, J. T. Wei, et al., Sexual health recovery after prostatectomy, external radiation, or brachytherapy for early stage prostate cancer, *Current Urology Reports* 5 (2004): 212–219.

15. E. J. Schwartz, P. Wong, R. J. Graydon, Sildenafil preserves intracorporeal smooth muscle after radical retropubic prostatectomy, *Journal of Urology* 171 (2004): 771–774.

16. Walsh et al., Patient-reported urinary continence; Walsh and Worthington, *Dr. Patrick Walsh's Guide,* 330.

17. Stanford et al., Urinary and sexual function; Talcott et al., Patient-reported symptoms; Hu et al., Predicting quality of life.

18. Hollenbeck et al., Sexual health recovery.

19. M. S. Litwin, N. Sadetsky, D. J. Pasta, et al., Bowel function and bother after treatment for early stage prostate cancer: A longitudinal quality of life analysis from CaPSURE, *Journal of Urology* 172 (2004): 515–519.

20. Jaroff, The man's cancer.

21. K. A. Roehl, M. Han, C. G. Ramos, et al., Cancer progression and sur-

vival rates following anatomical radical retropubic prostatectomy in 3,478 consecutive patients: Long-term results, *Journal of Urology* 172 (2004): 910–914; H. B. Carter, J. I. Epstein, A. W. Partin, Influence of age and prostate-specific antigen on the chance of curable prostate cancer among men with nonpalpable disease, *Urology* 53 (1999): 126–130.

22. M. B. Gretzer, J. I. Epstein, C. R. Pound, et al., Substratification of stage T1c prostate cancer based on the probability of biochemical recurrence, *Urology* 60 (2002): 1034–39; G. P. Swanson, M. W. Riggs, J. D. Earle, et al., Long-term follow-up of radical retropubic prostatectomy for prostate cancer, *European Urology* 42 (2002): 212–216.

23. G. W. Hull, F. Rabbani, F. Abbas, et al., Cancer control with radical prostatectomy alone in 1,000 consecutive patients, *Journal of Urology* 67 (2002): 528–534; Roehl et al., Cancer progression and survival rates; H. Zincke, J. E. Oesterling, M. L. Blute, et al., Long-term (15 years) results after radical prostatectomy for clinically localized (stage T2c or lower) prostate cancer, *Journal of Urology* 152 (1994): 1850–57; M. Han, A. W. Partin, C. R. Pound, et al., Long-term biochemical disease-free and cancer-specific survival following anatomic radical retropubic prostatectomy, *Urologic Clinics of North America* 28 (2001): 555–565; M. S. Litwin, D. P. Lubeck, G. M. Spitalny, et al., Mental health in men treated for early stage prostate carcinoma: A posttreatment, longitudinal quality of life analysis from the Cancer of the Prostate Strategic Urologic Research Endeavor, *Cancer* 95 (2002): 54–60.

4. Radiation Treatment

1. S. R. Denmeade and J. T. Isaacs, Development of prostate cancer treatment: The good news, *Prostate* 58 (2004): 211–224.

2. Peter D. Grimm, John C. Blasko, and John E. Sylvester (eds.), *The Prostate Cancer Treatment Book* (New York: McGraw Hill, 2004), 113; Denmeade and Isaacs, Development of prostate cancer treatment.

3. W. W. Wong, S. E. Schild, S. A. Vora, et al., Association of percent positive prostate biopsies and perineural invasion with biochemical outcome after external beam radiotherapy for localized prostate cancer, *International Journal of Radiation Oncology, Biology, Physics* 60 (2004): 24–29.

4. S. M. Alibhai, M. D. Krahn, M. M. Cohen, et al., Is there age bias in the treatment of localized prostate carcinoma? *Cancer* 100 (2004): 72–81.

5. M. Bolla, H. van Poppel, P. van Cangh, et al., Postoperative radiotherapy after radical prostatectomy: A randomized controlled trial (EORTC trial 22911), *Lancet* 366 (2005): 572–578.

6. Phyllis M. Windsor, Kathleen F. Nicol, Joan Potter, A randomized, controlled trial of aerobic exercise for treatment-related fatigue in men receiving radical external beam radiotherapy for localized prostate carcinoma, *Cancer* 101 (2004): 550–557.

7. I. Staff, A. Salner, R. Bohannon, et al., Disease-specific symptoms and

general quality of life of patients with prostate carcinoma before and after primary three-dimensional conformal radiotherapy, *Cancer* 98 (2003): 2335–43; D. F. Penson and M. S. Litwin, The physical burden of prostate cancer, *Urologic Clinics of North America* 30 (2003): 305–313; B. G. Gardner, A. L. Zietman, W. U. Shipley, et al., Late normal tissue sequelae in the second decade after high dose radiation therapy with combined photons and conformal protons for locally advanced prostate cancer, *Journal of Urology* 167 (2002): 123–126.

8. J. T. Wei, R. L. Dunn, H. M. Sandler, et al., Comprehensive comparison of health-related quality of life after contemporary therapies for localized prostate cancer, *Journal of Clinical Oncology* 20 (2002): 557–566; J. A. Talcott, J. A. Clark, P. C. Stark, Long-term treatment related complications of brachytherapy for early prostate cancer: A survey of patients previously treated, *Journal of Urology* 166 (2001): 494–499; M. S. Litwin, J. M. Brandeis, C. M. Burnison, et al., Quality of life outcomes after brachytherapy for early prostate cancer, *Prostate Cancer and Prostatic Diseases* 2 (suppl. 3) (1999): S19–S20.

9. A. L. Potosky, W. W. Davis, R. M. Hoffman, et al., Five-year outcomes after prostatectomy or radiotherapy for prostate cancer: The Prostate Cancer Outcomes Study, *Journal of the National Cancer Institute* 96 (2004): 1358–67.

10. Potosky et al., Five-year outcomes; C. A. Mantz, P. Song, E. Farhangi, et al., Potency probability following conformal megavoltage radiotherapy using conventional doses for localized prostate cancer, *International Journal of Radiation Oncology, Biology, Physics* 37 (1997): 551–557; Staff et al., Disease-specific symptoms; M. S. Litwin, S. C. Flanders, D. J. Pasta, et al., Sexual function and bother after radical prostatectomy or radiation for prostate cancer: Multivariate quality-of-life analysis from CaPSURE, *Urology* 54 (1999): 503–508; Talcott et al., Long-term treatment related complications; T. M. Downs, N. Sadetsky, D. J. Pasta, et al., Health related quality of life patterns in patients treated with interstitial prostate brachytherapy for localized prostate cancer—data from CaPSURE, *Journal of Urology* 170 (2003): 1822–27; G. Finney, A.-M. Haynes, P. Cross, et al., Cross-sectional analysis of sexual function after prostate brachytherapy, *Urology* 66 (2005): 377–381; Wei et al., Comprehensive comparison; B. K. Hollenbeck, R. L. Dunn, J. T. Wei, et al., Sexual health recovery after prostatectomy, external radiation, or brachytherapy for early stage prostate cancer, *Current Urology Reports* 5 (2004): 212–219; L. R. Schover, R. T. Fouladi, C. L. Warneke, et al., Defining sexual outcomes after treatment for localized prostate carcinoma, *Cancer* 95 (2002): 1773–85; I. S. Grills, A. A. Martinez, M. Hollander, et al., High dose rate brachytherapy as prostate cancer monotherapy reduces toxicity compared to low dose rate palladium seeds, *Journal of Urology* 171 (2004): 1098–1104.

11. Staff et al., Disease-specific symptoms; Potosky et al., Five-year outcomes; Gardner et al., Late normal tissue sequelae.

12. N. N. Baxter, J. E. Tepper, S. B. Durham, et al., Increased risk of rectal

cancer after prostate radiation: A population-based study, *Gastroenterology* 128 (2005): 819–824.

13. Talcott et al., Long-term treatment related complications; M. S. Litwin, N. Sadetsky, D. J. Pasta, et al., Bowel function and bother after treatment for early stage prostate cancer: A longitudinal quality of life analysis from CaPSURE, *Journal of Urology* 172 (2004): 515–519; Wei et al., Comprehensive comparison.

14. M. J. Zelefsky, Z. Fuks, M. Hunt, et al., High dose radiation delivered by intensity modulated conformal radiotherapy improves the outcome of localized prostate cancer, *Journal of Urology* 166 (2001): 876–881.

15. A. L. Hanlon, H. Diratzouian, G. E. Hanks, et al., Posttreatment prostate-specific antigen nadir highly predictive of distant failure and death from prostate cancer, *International Journal of Radiation Oncology, Biology, Physics* 53 (2002): 297–303; F. A. Critz, A standard definition of disease freedom is needed for prostate cancer: Undetectable prostate specific antigen compared with the American Society of Therapeutic Radiology and Oncology consensus definition, *Journal of Urology* 167 (2002): 1310–13.

16. A. V. D'Amico, A. A. Renshaw, B. Sussman, et al., Pretreatment PSA velocity and risk of death from prostate cancer following external beam radiation therapy, *Journal of the American Medical Association* 294 (2005): 440–447.

17. J. C. Hu, L. Kwan, C. S. Saigal, et al., Regret in men treated for localized prostate cancer, *Journal of Urology* 169 (2003): 2279–83.

5. Hormone Treatment

1. M. R. Cooperberg, G. D. Grossfeld, D. P. Lubeck, et al., National practice patterns and time trends in androgen ablation for localized prostate cancer, *Journal of the National Cancer Institute* 95 (2003): 981–989.

2. M. Peyromaure, N. B. Delongchamps, B. Debré, et al., Intermittent androgen deprivation for biologic recurrence after radical prostatectomy: Long-term experience, *Urology* 65 (2005): 724–729.

3. H. W. Daniell, S. R. Dunn, D. W. Ferguson, et al., Progressive osteoporosis during androgen deprivation therapy for prostate cancer, *Journal of Urology* 163 (2000): 181–186; V. B. Shahinian, Y.-F. Kuo, J. L. Freeman, et al., Risk of fracture after androgen deprivation for prostate cancer, *New England Journal of Medicine* 352 (2005): 154–164.

4. E. Salminen, R. Portin, J. Korpela, et al., Androgen deprivation and cognition in prostate cancer, *British Journal of Cancer* 89 (2003): 971–976.

5. M. Bolla, L. Collette, L. Blank, et al., Long-term results with immediate androgen suppression and external irradiation in patients with locally advanced prostate cancer (an EORTC study): A phase III randomised trial, *Lancet* 360 (2002): 103–108.

6. C. A. Lawton, K. Winter, K. Murray, et al., Updated results of the

Phase III Radiation Therapy Oncology Group (RTOG) Trial 85-31 evaluating the potential benefit of androgen suppression following standard radiation therapy for unfavorable prognosis carcinoma of the prostate, *International Journal of Radiation Oncology, Biology, Physics* 49 (2001): 937–946; M. V. Pilepich, K. Winter, M. J. John, et al., Phase III Radiation Therapy Oncology Group (RTOG) Trial 86-10 of androgen deprivation adjuvant to definitive radiotherapy in locally advanced carcinoma of the prostate, *International Journal of Radiation Oncology, Biology, Physics* 50 (2001): 1243–52; G. E. Hanks, T. F. Pajak, A. Porter, et al., Phase III trial of long-term adjuvant androgen deprivation after neoadjuvant hormonal cytoreduction and radiotherapy in locally advanced carcinoma of the prostate: The Radiation Therapy Outcome Group Protocol 92-02, *Journal of Clinical Oncology* 21 (2003): 3972–78; A. V. D'Amico, J. Manola, M. Loffredo, et al., 6-month androgen suppression plus radiation therapy vs radiation therapy alone for patients with clinically localized prostate cancer, *Journal of the American Medical Association* 292 (2004): 821–827.

7. J. W. Moul, J. Anderson, D. F. Penson, et al., Early prostate cancer: Prevention, treatment modalities, and quality of life issues, *European Urology* 44 (2003): 283–293; W. A. See, M. P. Wirth, D. G. McLeod, et al., Bicalutamide as immediate therapy either alone or as adjuvant to standard care of patients with localized or locally advanced prostate cancer: First analysis of the early prostate cancer program, *Journal of Urology* 168 (2002): 429–435.

8. M. S. Soloway, K. Pareek, R. Sharifi, et al., Neoadjuvant androgen ablation before radical prostatectomy in cT2bNxM0 prostate cancer: 5-year results, *Journal of Urology* 167 (2002): 112–116; Cooperberg et al., National practice patterns.

6. Cryotherapy

1. P. Perrotte, M. S. Litwin, E. J. McGuire, et al., Quality of life after salvage cryotherapy: The impact of treatment parameters, *Journal of Urology* 162 (1999): 398–402; K.-R. Han, J. K. Cohen, R. J. Miller, et al., Treatment of organ confined prostate cancer with third generation cryosurgery: Preliminary multicenter experience, *Journal of Urology* 170 (2003): 1126–30; K. Shinohara, Prostate cancer: Cryotherapy, *Urologic Clinics of North America* 30 (2003): 725–736.

2. J. P. Long, D. Bahn, F. Lee, et al., Five-year retrospective, multi-institutional pooled analysis of cancer-related outcomes after cryosurgical ablation of the prostate, *Urology* 57 (2001): 518–523; D. K. Bahn, F. Lee, R. Badalament, et al., Targeted cryoablation of the prostate: 7-year outcomes in the primary treatment of prostate cancer, *Urology* 60 (2 suppl. 1) (2002): 3–11.

7. Alternative and Experimental Therapies

1. M. C. Lippert, R. McClain, J. C. Boyd, et al., Alternative medicine use in patients with localized prostate carcinoma treated with curative intent, *Cancer* 86 (1999): 2642–48.

2. J. D. Hall, E. A. Bissonette, J. C. Boyd, et al., Motivations and influences on the use of complementary medicine in patients with localized prostate cancer treated with curative intent: Results of a pilot study, *BJU International* 91 (2003): 603–607; S. Wilkinson, L. G. Gomella, J. A. Smith, et al., Attitudes and use of complementary medicine in men with prostate cancer, *Journal of Urology* 168 (2002): 2505–9; A. Barqawi, E. Gamito, C. O'Donnell, et al., Herbal and vitamin supplement use in a prostate cancer screening population, *Urology* 63 (2004): 288–292; R. K. Nam, N. Fleshner, E. Rakovitch, et al., Prevalence and patterns of the use of complementary therapies among prostate cancer patients: An epidemiological analysis, *Journal of Urology* 161 (1999): 1521–24.

3. Saw palmetto for benign prostatic hyperplasia, *Medical Letter* 41 (1999): 18.

4. H. Boon, K. Westlake, M. Stewart, et al., Use of complementary/alternative medicine by men diagnosed with prostate cancer: Prevalence and characteristics, *Urology* 62 (2003): 849–853; J. Eng, D. Ramsum, M. Verhoef, et al., A population-based survey of complementary and alternative medicine use in men recently diagnosed with prostate cancer, *Integrative Cancer Therapies* 2 (2003); 212–216; Wilkinson et al., Attitudes and use of complementary medicine; J. L. Beebe-Dimmer, D. P. Wood Jr., S. B. Gruber, et al., Use of complementary and alternative medicine in men with family history of prostate cancer: A pilot study, *Urology* 63 (2004): 282–287.

5. M. M. Lee, J. S. Chang, B. Jacobs, et al., Complementary and alternative medicine use among men with prostate cancer in 4 ethnic populations, *American Journal of Public Health* 92 (2002): 1606–9.

6. D. Schardt, Urine trouble, *Nutrition Action Healthletter,* December 2003, 7–9; R. S. Ranga, R. Girija, M. Nur-e-alam, et al., Rasagenthi lehyam (RL) a novel complementary and alternative medicine for prostate cancer, *Cancer Chemotherapy and Pharmacology* 54 (2004): 7–15.

7. Wilkinson et al., Attitudes and use of complementary medicine; Nam et al., Prevalence and patterns; D. R. Miller, G. T. Anderson, J. J. Stark, et al., Phase I/II trial of the safety and efficacy of shark cartilage in the treatment of advanced cancer, *Journal of Clinical Oncology* 16 (1998): 3649–55.

8. M. P. Kosty, PC-SPES: Hope or hype? *Journal of Clinical Oncology* 22 (2004): 3657–59; James Lewis, *The Herbal Remedy for Prostate Cancer* (Westbury, N.Y.: Health Education Literary Publisher, 1999), 41.

9. Lewis, *The Herbal Remedy,* 102.

10. Ibid., vi.

11. W. K. Oh and E. J. Small, Complementary and alternative therapies in prostate cancer, *Seminars in Oncology* 29 (2002): 575–584; J. Gillis, Herbal remedies turn deadly for patients, *Washington Post,* September 5, 2004.

12. Kosty, PC-SPES: hope or hype?; 3657; Gillis, Herbal remedies turn deadly.

13. Gillis, Herbal remedies turn deadly.

14. W. K. Oh, P. W. Kantoff, V. Weinberg, et al., Prospective, multicenter, randomized phase II trial of the herbal supplement, PC-SPES, and diethylstilbestrol in patients with androgen-independent prostate cancer, *Journal of Clinical Oncology* 22 (2004): 3705–12; Gillis, Herbal remedies turn deadly.

15. Gillis, Herbal remedies turn deadly.

8. Treatment Decisions

1. Quoted in A. Grove, Taking on prostate cancer, *Fortune,* May 13, 1996.

2. M. Overmyer, Tx delay raises risk in patients with high-risk PCa, *Urology Times,* May 1, 2004.

3. J.-E. Johansson, H.-O. Adami, S.-O. Andersson, et al., High 10-year survival rate in patients with early, untreated prostatic cancer, *Journal of the American Medical Association* 267 (1992): 2191–96; J.-E. Johansson, O. Andrén, S.-O. Andersson, et al., Natural history of early, localized prostate cancer, *Journal of the American Medical Association* 291 (2004): 2713–19.

4. Johansson et al., Natural history.

5. L. Holmberg, A. Bill-Axelson, F. Helgesen, et al., A randomized trial comparing radical prostatectomy with watchful waiting in early prostate cancer, *New England Journal of Medicine* 347 (2002): 781–789.

6. G. W. Chodak, R. A. Thisted, G. S. Gerber, et al., Results of conservative management of clinically localized prostate cancer, *New England Journal of Medicine* 330 (1994): 242–248.

7. P. C. Albertsen, J. A. Hanley, and J. Fine, 20-year outcomes following conservative management of clinically localized prostate cancer, *Journal of the American Medical Association* 293 (2005): 2095–2101.

8. G. Steineck, F. Helgesen, J. Adolfsson, et al., Quality of life after radical prostatectomy or watchful waiting, *New England Journal of Medicine* 347 (2002): 790–796; M. Jønler, O. S. Nielsen, and H. Wolf, Urinary symptoms, potency, and quality of life in patients with localized prostate cancer followed up with deferred treatment, *Urology* 52 (1998): 1055–62; S. A. Arredondo, T. M. Downs, D. P. Lubeck, et al., Watchful waiting and health related quality of life for patients with localized prostate cancer: Data from CaPSURE, *Journal of Urology* 172 (2004): 1830–34.

9. E. M. Messing and I. Thompson Jr., Follow-up of conservatively managed prostate cancer: Watchful waiting and primary hormonal therapy, *Urologic Clinics of North America* 30 (2003): 687–702; D. Ornish, G. Weidner, W. R. Fair, et al., Intensive lifestyle changes may affect the progression of prostate cancer, *Journal of Urology* 174 (2005): 1065–70.

10. Leon Jaroff, The man's cancer, *Time,* April 1, 1996; M. R. Cooperberg, J. M. Broering, D. M. Latini, et al., Patterns of practice in the United States: Insights from CaPSURE on prostate cancer management, *Current Urology Reports* 5 (2004): 166–172; S. R. Harlan, M. R. Cooperberg, E. P. Elkin, et al., Time trends and characteristics of men choosing watchful waiting for initial treatment of localized prostate cancer: Results from CaPSURE, *Journal of Urology* 170 (2003): 1804–7.

11. H. Wu, L. Sun, J. W. Moul, et al., Watchful waiting and factors predictive of secondary treatment of localized prostate cancer, *Journal of Urology* 171 (2004): 1111–16.

12. Patrick C. Walsh and Janet F. Worthington, *Dr. Patrick Walsh's Guide to Surviving Prostate Cancer* (New York: Time Warner, 2001), 184; Aubrey Pilgrim, *A Revolutionary Approach to Prostate Cancer* (Pittsburgh: Sterling House, 1997), 97; J. A. Kaswick, Whitmorisms [letter], *Urology* 64 (2004): 189.

13. C. Bankhead, Still waiting on watchful waiting: Clinical trials test surveillance, *Journal of the National Cancer Institute* 95 (2003): 1657–59; C. A. Carter, T. Donahue, L. Sun, et al., Temporarily deferred therapy (watchful waiting) for men younger than 70 years and with low-risk localized prostate cancer in the prostate-specific antigen era, *Journal of Clinical Oncology* 21 (2003): 4001–8; M. I. Patel, D. T. DeConcini, E. Lopez-Corona, et al., An analysis of men with clinically localized prostate cancer who deferred definitive therapy, *Journal of Urology* 171 (2004): 1520–24.

14. A. Peeters, J. J. Barendregt, F. Willekens, et al., Obesity in adulthood and its consequences for life expectancy: A life-table analysis, *Annals of Internal Medicine* 138 (2003): 24–32.

15. Jaroff, The man's cancer.

16. S. S. Mehta, D. P. Lubeck, D. J. Pasta, et al., Fear of cancer recurrence in patients undergoing definitive treatment for prostate cancer: Results from CaPSURE, *Journal of Urology* 170 (2003): 1931–33; M. S. Litwin, D. P. Lubeck, G. M. Spitalny, et al., Mental health in men treated for early stage prostate carcinoma: A posttreatment, longitudinal quality of life analysis from the Cancer of the Prostate Strategic Urologic Research Endeavor, *Cancer* 95 (2002): 54–60.

17. L. R. Schover, R. T. Fouladi, C. L. Warneke, et al., Defining sexual outcomes after treatment for localized prostate cancinoma, *Cancer* 95 (2002): 1773–85.

18. B. K. Hollenbeck, R. L. Dunn, J. T. Wei, et al., Sexual health recovery after prostatectomy, external radiation, or brachytherapy for early stage prostate cancer, *Current Urology Reports* 5 (2004): 212–219; D. F. Penson, M. S. Litwin, and N. K. Aaronson, Health related quality of life in men with prostate cancer, *Journal of Urology* 169 (2003): 1653–61; J. M. Brandeis, M. S. Litwin, C. M. Burnison, et al., Quality of life outcomes after brachytherapy for early stage prostate cancer, *Journal of Urology* 163 (2000): 851–857; H. Borchers, R. Kirschner-Hermanns, B. Brehmer, et al., Permanent 125I-seed

brachytherapy or radical prostatectomy: A prospective comparison considering oncological and quality of life results, *BJU International* 94 (2004): 805–811.

19. A. L. Potosky, W. W. Davis, R. M. Hoffman, et al., Five-year outcomes after prostatectomy or radiotherapy for prostate cancer: The Prostate Cancer Outcomes Study, *Journal of the National Cancer Institute* 96 (2004): 1358–67.

20. E. B. Bradley, E. A. Bissonette, and D. Theodorescu, Determinants of long-term quality of life and voiding function of patients treated with radical prostatectomy or permanent brachytherapy for prostate cancer, *BJU International* 94 (2004): 1003–9; J. T. Wei, R. L. Dunn, H. M. Sandler, et al., Comprehensive comparison of health-related quality of life after contemporary therapies for localized prostate cancer, *Journal of Clinical Oncology* 20 (2002): 557–566.

21. Hollenbeck et al., Sexual health recovery.

22. Walsh and Worthington, *Dr. Patrick Walsh's Guide,* 211; P. C. Walsh, P. Marschke, D. Ricker, et al., Patient-reported urinary continence and sexual function after anatomic radical prostatectomy, *Urology* 55 (2000): 58–61; Schover et al., Defining sexual outcomes.

23. F. J. Fowler Jr., M. J. Barry, G. Lu-Yao, et al., Effect of radical prostatectomy for prostate cancer on patient quality of life: Results from a Medicare survey, *Urology* 45 (1995): 1007–15.

24. Penson et al., Health related quality of life; J. A. Talcott, P. Rieker, J. A. Clark, et al., Patient-reported symptoms after primary therapy for early prostate cancer: Results of a prospective cohort study, *Journal of Clinical Oncology* 16 (1998): 275–283; Potosky et al., Five-year outcomes; Wei et al., Comprehensive comparison; M. S. Litwin, D. J. Pasta, J. Yu, et al., Urinary function and bother after radical prostatectomy or radiation for prostate cancer: A longitudinal multivariate quality of life analysis from the Cancer of the Prostate Strategic Urologic Research Endeavor, *Journal of Urology* 164 (2000): 1973–77.

25. Wei et al., Comprehensive comparison.

26. Ibid.; Talcott et al., Patient-reported symptoms; Penson, Litwin, and Aaronson, Health related quality of life; Potosky et al., Five-year outcomes; M. S. Litwin, N. Sadetsky, D. J. Pasta, et al., Bowel function and bother after treatment for early stage prostate cancer: A longitudinal quality of life analysis from CaPSURE, *Journal of Urology* 172 (2004): 515–519.

27. David G. Bostwick, E. David Crawford, Celestia S. Higano, et al. (eds.), *American Cancer Society's Complete Guide to Prostate Cancer* (Atlanta: American Cancer Society, 2005), 85.

28. C. B. Begg, E. R. Riedel, P. B. Bach, et al., Variations in morbidity after radical prostatectomy, *New England Journal of Medicine* 346 (2002): 1138–44; F. J. Bianco Jr., E. R. Riedel, C. B. Begg, et al., Variations among high volume surgeons in the rate of complications after radical prostatectomy: Further evidence that technique matters, *Journal of Urology* 173 (2005): 2099–2103; K. A. Roehl, M. Han, C. G. Ramos, et al., Cancer progression and survival

rates following anatomical radical retropubic prostatectomy in 3,478 consecutive patients: Long-term results, *Journal of Urology* 172 (2004): 910–914; M. Han, A. W. Partin, C. R. Pound, et al., Long-term biochemical disease-free and cancer-specific survival, *Urologic Clinics of North America* 28 (2001): 555–565; G. W. Hull, F. Rabbani, F. Abbas, et al., Cancer control with radical prostatectomy alone in 1,000 consecutive patients, *Journal of Urology* 167 (2002): 528–534.

29. J. Brandeis, C. L. Pashos, J. M. Henning, et al., A nationwide charge comparison of the principal treatments for early stage prostate carcinoma, *Cancer* 89 (2000): 1792–99.

30. C. S. Saigal and M. S. Litwin, The economic costs of early stage prostate cancer, *Pharmacoeconomics* 20 (2002): 869–878.

31. Michael A. Dorso, *Seeds of Hope: A Physician's Personal Triumph over Prostate Cancer* (Battle Creek, Mich.: Acorn Publishing, 2000), 100–101.

9. Your Support System

1. M. D. Llorente, M. Burke, G. R. Gregory, et al., Prostate cancer: A significant risk factor for late-life suicide, *American Journal of Geriatric Psychiatry* 13 (2005): 195–201.

2. Richard Y. Handy, *Confronting the Emotional and Physical Challenges of Prostate Cancer* (Amherst, N.Y.: Prometheus Books, 1996), 168.

3. Cornelius Ryan and Kathryn Morgan Ryan, *A Private Battle* (New York: Simon and Schuster, 1979), 20; Anatole Broyard, *Intoxicated by My Illness* (New York: Ballantine Books, 1992), 29.

4. Handy, *Confronting the Challenges,* 43.

5. Ryan and Ryan, *A Private Battle,* 43.

6. Desiree Howe, *His Prostate and Me* (Houston: Winedale Publishing, 2002), 104.

7. Barbara Wainrib and Sandra Haber, *Men, Women, and Prostate Cancer* (Oakland, Calif.: New Harbinger, 2000), 231.

8. David Seifman, *New York Post,* December 12, 2000.

9. Jeff M. Michalski and John E. Sylvester, What part do spouses and partners play?, in Peter D. Grimm, John C. Blasko, and John E. Sylvester (eds.), *The Prostate Cancer Treatment Book* (New York: McGraw Hill, 2004), 61.

10. Katie Hafner, Treated for illness, then lost in labyrinth of bills, *New York Times,* October 13, 2005.

11. A. Krongard, H. Lai, M. A. Burke, et al., Marriage and mortality in prostate cancer, *Journal of Urology* 156 (1996): 1696–1700.

12. J. Harden, A. Schafenacker, L. Northouse, et al., Couples' experiences with prostate cancer: Focus group research, *Oncology Nursing Forum* 29 (2002): 701–709; Ryan and Ryan, *A Private Battle,* 37.

13. R. J. Volk, S. B. Cantor, A. R. Cass, et al., Preferences of husbands and wives for outcome of prostate cancer screening and treatment, *Journal of General Internal Medicine* 19 (2004): 339–348.

14. T. O. Blank, Gay men and prostate cancer: Invisible diversity, *Journal of Clinical Oncology* 23 (2005): 2593–96.

15. Broyard, *Intoxicated by My Illness,* 44.

16. Ryan and Ryan, *A Private Battle,* 119; Handy, *Confronting the Challenges,* 58–59; Michael Korda, *Man to Man: Surviving Prostate Cancer* (New York: Vintage Books, 1996), 186; Audrey Currie Newton, *Living with Prostate Cancer* (Toronto: McClelland and Stewart, 1996), 90.

17. C. J. Bradley, D. Neumark, Z. Luo, et al., Employment outcomes of men treated for prostate cancer, *Journal of the National Cancer Institute* 97 (2005): 958–965.

18. Handy, *Confronting the Challenges,* 40.

10. Major Complications and Their Treatment

1. Anatole Broyard, *Intoxicated by My Illness* (New York: Ballantine Books, 1992), 28.

2. Patrick C. Walsh and Janet F. Worthington, *Dr. Patrick Walsh's Guide to Surviving Prostate Cancer* (New York: Time Warner, 2001), 244; Charles R. Williams and Vernon A. Williams, *That Black Men Might Live* (Roscoe, Ill.: Hilton Publishing, 2003), 42; J. A. Smith Jr., Sexual function after radical prostatectomy (editorial), *Journal of Urology* 169 (2003): 1465.

3. Walsh and Worthington, *Dr. Patrick Walsh's Guide,* 247; Sheldon Marks, *Prostate and Cancer: A Family Guide to Diagnosis, Treatment, and Survival,* 3rd ed. (New York: Perseus, 2003), 227.

4. Marks, *Prostate and Cancer,* 227; Aubrey Pilgrim, *A Revolutionary Approach to Prostate Cancer* (Pittsburgh: SterlingHouse, 1997), 213; Daniel W. Nixon and Max Gomez, *The Prostate Health Program: A Guide to Preventing and Controlling Prostate Cancer* (New York: Free Press, 2004), 162; Treatment for urinary incontinence among prostate cancer surgery patients, *Medical News Today,* October 19, 2004.

5. S. Namiki, S. Saito, S. Ishidoya, et al., Adverse effect of radical prostatectomy on nocturia and voiding frequency symptoms, *Urology* 66 (2005): 147–151.

6. William Martin, *My Prostate and Me* (New York: Cadell and Davies, 1994), 125–127; Walsh and Worthington, *Dr. Patrick Walsh's Guide,* 251, 326.

7. Leon Prochnik, *You Can't Make Love if You're Dead* (Los Angeles: Ari Press, 2000), 117; Bert Gottlieb and Thomas J. Mawn, *The Men's Club: How to Lose Your Prostate Without Losing Your Sense of Humor* (Oxnard, Calif.: Pathfinder Publishing, 1999), 34; Martin, *My Prostate and Me,* 127.

8. Male orgasmic quality affected by prostate cancer surgery, *Medical News Today,* May 9, 2004, Michael A. Dorso, *Seeds of Hope: A Physician's Personal Triumph over Prostate Cancer* (Battle Creek, Mich.: Acorn Publishing, 2000), 227.

9. Charles Neider, *Adam's Burden: An Explorer's Personal Odyssey Through Prostate Cancer* (Lanham, Md.: Madison Books, 2001), 13.

10. Walsh and Worthington, *Dr. Patrick Walsh's Guide,* 330.

11. D. F. Penson, D. McLerran, Z. Feng, et al., 5-Year urinary and sexual outcomes after radical prostatectomy: Results from the Prostate Cancer Outcomes Study, *Journal of Urology* 173 (2005): 1701–5; C. A. Holden, R. I. McLachlan, M. Pitts, et al., Men in Australia Telephone Survey (MATeS): A national survey of the reproductive health and concerns of middle-aged and older Australian men, *Lancet* 366 (2005): 218–224.

12. M. C. Haffner, P. K. Landis, C. S. Saigal, et al., Health-related quality-of-life outcomes after anatomic retropubic radical prostatectomy in the phosphodiesterase type 5 era: Impact of neurovascular bundle preservation, *Urology* 66 (2005): 371–376.

13. B. G. Bokhour, J. A. Clark, T. S. Inui, et al., Sexuality after treatment for early prostate cancer: Exploring the meanings of "erectile dysfunction," *Journal of General Internal Medicine* 16 (2001): 649–655.

14. Daniel W. Nixon and Max Gomez, *The Prostate Health Program: A Guide to Preventing and Controlling Prostate Cancer* (New York: Free Press, 2004), 171.

15. Dorso, *Seeds of Hope,* 199–200.

16. Ralph Alterowitz and Barbara Alterowitz, *The Lovin' Ain't Over: The Couples Guide to Better Sex after Prostate Disease* (Westbury, N.Y.: Health Education Literary Publisher, 1999), 47.

17. Ibid., 7, 39; Dorso, *Seeds of Hope,* 69, 193.

18. Penson et al., 5-Year urinary and sexual outcomes.

19. Viagra and loss of vision, *Medical Letter* 47 (2005): 49; R. Akash, D. Hrishikesh, P. Amith, et al., Association of combined nonarteritic anterior ischemic optic neuropathy (NAION) and obstruction of cilioretinal artery with overdose of Viagra, *Journal of Ocular Pharmacology and Therpeutics* 21 (2005): 315–317.

20. E. J. Schwartz, P. Wong, and R. J. Graydon, Sildenafil preserves intra-corporeal smooth muscle after radical retropubic prostatectomy, *Journal of Urology* 171 (2004): 771–774.

21. Walsh and Worthington, *Dr. Patrick Walsh's Guide,* 344.

22. Neider, *Adam's Burden,* 157.

23. A. L. Burnett, Erectile dysfunction following radical prostatectomy, *Journal of the American Medical Association* 293 (2005): 2648–53.

11. What Happens if the Cancer Spreads or Comes Back?

1. Joseph Osterling, preface, in Joseph E. Osterling and Mark A. Moyad, *The ABCs of Prostate Cancer: The Book That Could Save Your Life* (Lanham, Md.: Madison Books, 1997).

2. M. Han, A. W. Partin, C. R. Pound, et al., Long-term biochemical

disease-free and cancer-specific survival, *Urologic Clinics of North America* 28 (2001): 555–565; C. M. Gonzalez, K. A. Roehl, J. A. V. Antenor, et al., Preoperative PSA level significantly associated with interval to biochemical progression after radical retropubic prostatectomy, *Urology* 64 (2004): 723–728; M. A. Khan, A. W. Partin, L. A. Mangold, et al., Probability of biochemical recurrence by analysis of pathologic stage, Gleason score, and margin status for localized prostate cancer, *Urology* 62 (2003): 866–871; C. G. Ramos, K. A. Roehl, J. A. V. Antenor, et al., Percent carcinoma in prostatectomy specimen is associated with risk of recurrence after radical prostatectomy in patients with pathologically organ confined prostate cancer, *Journal of Urology* 172 (2004): 137–140.

3. M. L. Blute, E. J. Bergstralh, A. Iocca, et al., Use of Gleason score, prostate specific antigen, seminal vesicle and margin status to predict biochemical failure after radical prostatectomy, *Journal of Urology* 165 (2001): 119–125.

4. M. W. Kattan, T. M. Wheeler, and P. T. Scardino, Postoperative nomogram for disease recurrence after radical prostatectomy for prostate cancer, *Journal of Clinical Oncology* 17 (1999): 1499–1507.

5. Patrick C. Walsh and Janet F. Worthington, *Dr. Patrick Walsh's Guide to Surviving Prostate Cancer* (New York: Time Warner, 2001), 294; S. J. Freedland, E. B. Humphreys, L. A. Mangold, et al., Risk of prostate cancer–specific mortality following biochemical recurrence after radical prostatectomy, *Journal of the American Medical Association* 294 (2005): 433–439.

6. J. B. Nelson and H. Lepor, Prostate cancer: Radical prostatectomy, *Urologic Clinics of North America* 30 (2003): 703–723.

7. C. R. Pound, A. W. Partin, M. A. Eisenberger, et al., Natural history of progression after PSA elevation following radical prostatectomy, *Journal of the American Medical Association* 281 (1999): 1591–97.

8. H. I. Scher, Management of prostate cancer after prostatectomy: Treating the patient, not the PSA [editorial], *Journal of the American Medical Association* 281 (1999): 1642–45.

9. J. Holzbeierlein, R. Payne, J. Weigel, et al., Long-term followup of metastatic prostate cancer, *Journal of Urology* 171 (2004): 2377.

10. M. G. Oefelein, V. S. Ricchiuti, P. W. Conrad, et al., Clinical predictors of androgen-independent prostate cancer and survival in the prostate-specific antigen era, *Urology* 60 (2002): 120–124.

11. Medical Research Council Prostate Cancer Working Party Investigators Group, Immediate versus deferred treatment for advanced prostatic cancer: Initial results of the Medical Research Council trial, *British Journal of Urology* 79 (1997): 235–246; E. M. Messing, J. Manola, M. Sarosdy, et al., Immediate hormonal therapy compared with observation after radical prostatectomy and pelvic lymphadenectomy in men with node-positive prostate cancer, *New England Journal of Medicine* 341 (1999): 1781–88.

12. Walsh and Worthington, *Dr. Patrick Walsh's Guide,* 372.

13. J. de Leval, P. Boca, E. Youssef, et al., Intermittent versus continuous total androgen blockade in the treatment of patients with advanced hormone-naïve prostate cancer: Results of a prospective randomized multicenter trial, *Clinical Prostate Cancer* 1 (2002): 163–171; E. Youssef, S. Tekyi-Mensah, K. Hart, et al., Intermittent androgen deprivation for patients with recurrent/metastatic prostate cancer, *American Journal of Clinical Oncology* 26 (2003): e119–e123; T. M. Lane, W. Ansell, D. Farrugia, et al., Long-term outcomes in patients with prostate cancer managed with intermittent androgen suppression, *Urologia Internationalis* 73 (2004): 117–122; B. Hellerstedt, Hormonal therapy options for patients with a rising prostate-specific antigen level after primary treatment for prostate cancer, *Urology* 62 (2003) (suppl. 6B): 79–86.

14. Nelson and Lepor, Prostate cancer.

15. A. J. Stephenson, S. F. Shariat, M. J. Zelefsky, et al., Salvage radiotherapy for recurrent prostate cancer after radical prostatectomy, *Journal of the American Medical Association* 291 (2004): 1325–32; O. K. MacDonald, S. E. Schild, S. A. Vora, et al., Radiotherapy for men with isolated increase in serum prostate specific antigen after radical prostatectomy, *Journal of Urology* 170 (2003): 1833–37.

16. D. P. Petrylak, C. M. Tangen, M. H. A. Hussain, et al., Docetaxel and estramustine compared with mitoxantrone and prednisone for advanced refractory prostate cancer, *New England Journal of Medicine* 351 (2004): 1513–20; I. F. Tannock, R. de Wit, W. R. Berry, et al., Docetaxel plus prednisone or mitoxantrone plus prednisone for advanced prostate cancer, *New England Journal of Medicine* 351 (2004): 1502–12.

17. N. A. Dawson and S. F. Slovin, Novel approaches to treat asymptomatic, hormone-naïve patients with rising prostate-specific antigen after primary treatment for prostate cancer, *Urology* 62 (2003) (suppl. 6B): 102–118.

18. E. C. Skinner and L. M. Glode, High-risk localized prostate cancer: Primary surgery and adjuvant therapy, *Urologic Oncology* 21 (2003): 219–227.

19. M. S. Litwin, D. P. Lubeck, M. L. Stoddard, et al., Quality of life before death for men with prostate cancer: Results from the CaPSURE database, *Journal of Urology* 165 (2001): 871–875; G. Sandblom, P. Carlsson, K. Sennfält, et al., A population-based study of pain and quality of life during the year before death in men with prostate cancer, *British Journal of Cancer* 90 (2004): 1163–68.

20. G. Y. Melmed, L. Kwan, K. Reid, et al., Quality of life at the end of life: Trends in patients with metastatic prostate cancer, *Urology* 59 (2002): 103–109.

21. Anatole Broyard, *Intoxicated by My Illness* (New York: Ballantine Books, 1992), 25.

22. Cornelius Ryan and Kathryn Morgan Ryan, *A Private Battle* (New York: Simon and Schuster, 1979), 208.

23. Charles Neider, *Adam's Burden: An Explorer's Personal Odyssey Through Prostate Cancer* (Lanham, Md.: Madison Books, 2001), 33.

12. What Is Known About the Causes?

1. P. Boyle, G. Severi, and G. G. Giles, The epidemiology of prostate cancer, *Urologic Clinics of North America* 30 (2003): 209–217.

2. W. A. Sakr, G. P. Haas, B. F. Cassin, et al., The frequency of carcinoma and intraepithelial neoplasia of the prostate in young male patients, *Journal of Urology* 150 (1993): 379–385.

3. A. S. Whittemore, P. M. Cirillo, D. Feldman, et al., Prostate specific antigen levels in young adulthood predict prostate cancer risk: Results from a cohort of black and white Americans, *Journal of Urology* 174 (2005): 872–876.

4. A. W. Hsing, L. Tsao, and S. S. Devesa, International trends and patterns of prostate cancer incidence and mortality, *International Journal of Cancer* 85 (2000): 60–67.

5. D. B. French and L. A. Jones, Minority issues in prostate disease, *Medical Clinics of North America* 89 (2005): 805–816; K. E. Gaston, D. Kim, S. Singh, et al., Racial differences in androgen receptor protein expression in men with clinically localized prostate cancer, *Journal of Urology* 170 (2003): 990–993.

6. P. B. Bach, H. H. Pham, D. Schrag, et al., Primary care physicians who treat blacks and whites, *New England Journal of Medicine* 351 (2004): 575–584.

7. P. N. Brawn, E. H. Johnson, D. L. Kuhl, et al., Stage at presentation and survival of white and black patients with prostate carcinoma, *Cancer* 71 (1993): 2569–73; A. S. Robbins, A. S. Whittemore, and S. K. Van Den Eeden, Race, prostate cancer survival, and membership in a large health maintenance organization, *Journal of the National Cancer Institute* 90 (1998): 986–990.

8. E. F. Torrey, Malignant neoplasms among Alaskan natives: An epidemiological approach to cancer, *McGill Medical Journal* 31 (1962): 107–115; G. Ehrsam, A. Lanier, P. Holck, et al., Cancer mortality among Alaska natives, 1994–1998, *Alaska Medicine* 43 (2001): 50–60, 83; Cancer mortality among American Indians and Alaska natives—United States, 1994–1998, *Morbidity and Mortality Weekly Reports* 52 (2003): 704–707; E. Dewailly, G. Mulvad, H. S. Pedersen, et al., Inuit are protected against prostate cancer, *Cancer Epidemiology, Biomarkers, and Prevention* 12 (2003): 926–927; D. N. Paltoo and K. C. Chu, Patterns in cancer incidence among American Indians/Alaska natives, United States, 1992–1999, *Public Health Reports* 119 (2004): 443–451; T. Haldoresen and T. Tynes, Cancer in the Sami population of North Norway, 1970–1997, *European Journal of Cancer Prevention* 14 (2005): 63–68.

9. F. E. Glover Jr., D. S. Coffey, L. L. Douglas, et al., The epidemiology of prostate cancer in Jamaica, *Journal of Urology* 159 (1998): 1984–86.

10. E. O. Kehinde, The geography of prostate cancer and its treatment in Africa, *Cancer Surveys. Preventing Prostate Cancer: Screening versus Chemoprevention* (Cold Spring Harbor, N.Y.: Cold Spring Harbor Laboratory Press, 1995), 281–286; D. N. Osegbe, Prostate cancer in Nigerians: Facts and non-facts, *Journal of Urology* 157 (1997): 1340–43.

11. H. G. Sim and C. W. S. Cheng, Changing demography of prostate cancer in Asia, *European Journal of Cancer* 41 (2005): 834–845.

12. H. Shimizu, R. K. Ross, L. Bernstein, et al., Cancers of the prostate and breast among Japanese and white immigrants in Los Angeles County, *British Journal of Cancer* 63 (1991): 963–966; L. S. Cook, M. Goldoft, S. M. Schwartz, et al., Incidence of adenocarcinoma of the prostate in Asian immigrants to the United States and their descendants, *Journal of Urology* 161 (1999): 152–155; B. Jin, L. Turner, Z. Zhou, et al., Ethnicity and migration as determinants of human prostate size, *Journal of Clinical Endocrinology and Metabolism* 84 (1999): 3613–19.

13. D. J. Waters, G. J. Patronek, D. G. Bostwick, et al., Comparing the age at prostate cancer diagnosis in humans and dogs (letter), *Journal of the National Cancer Institute* 88 (1996): 1686–87.

14. S. O. Dalton, L. Mellemkjaer, L. Thomassen, et al., Risk for cancer in a cohort of patients hospitalized for schizophrenia in Denmark, 1969–1993, *Schizophrenia Research* 75 (2005): 315–324; A. Grinshpoon, M. Barchana, A. Ponizovsky, et al., Cancer in schizophrenia: Is the risk higher or lower? *Schizophrenia Research* 73 (2005): 333–341; P. B. Mortensen, Neuroleptic medication and reduced risk of prostate cancer in schizophrenic patients, *Acta Psychiatrica Scandinavica* 85 (1992): 390–393.

15. B. S. Carter, G. S. Bova, T. H. Beaty, et al., Hereditary prostate cancer: Epidemiologic and clinical features, *Journal of Urology* 150 (1993): 797–802.

16. A Bond of Brothers, *NEWSWISE Medical News,* September 2, 2004.

17. P. Lichtenstein, N. V. Holm, P. K. Verkasalo, et al., Environmental and heritable factors in the causation of cancer: Analyses of cohorts of twins from Sweden, Denmark, and Finland, *New England Journal of Medicine* 343 (2000): 78–85.

18. D. J. Schaid, The complex genetic epidemiology of prostate cancer, *Human Molecular Genetics* 13 (2004): R103–R121; K. Hemminki and X. Li, Association of brain tumours with other neoplasms in families, *European Journal of Cancer* 40 (2004): 253–259.

19. E. D. Crawford, Epidemiology of prostate cancer, *Journal of Urology* 62 (suppl. 6A) (2003): 3–12.

20. Y. M. Centifanto, H. E. Kaufman, Z. S. Zam, et al., Herpesvirus particles in prostatic carcinoma cells, *Journal of Virology* 12 (1973): 1608–11.

21. M. Samanta, L. Harkins, K. Klemm, et al., High prevalence of human cytomegalovirus in prostatic intraepithelial neoplasia and prostatic carcinoma, *Journal of Urology* 170 (2003): 998–1002; M. J. Leskinen, R. Vainion-paa, S. Syrjanen, et al., Herpes simplex virus, cytomegalovirus, and papillo-

mavirus DNA are not found in patients with chronic pelvic pain syndrome undergoing radical prostatectomy for localized prostate cancer, *Urology* 61 (2003): 397–401; S. Grinstein, M. V. Preciado, P. Gattuso, et al., Demonstration of Epstein-Barr virus in carcinomas of various sites, *Cancer Research* 62 (2002): 4876–78; L. J. Hoffman, C. H. Bunker, P. E. Pellett, et al., Elevated seroprevalence of human herpesvirus 8 among men with prostate cancer, *Journal of Infectious Diseases* 189 (2004): 15–20; F. Wang-Johanning, A. R. Frost, B. Jian, et al., Detecting the expression of human endogenous retrovirus E envelope transcripts in human prostate adenocarcinoma, *Cancer* 98 (2003): 187–197; A. Zambrano, M. Kalantari, and A. Simoneau, Detection of human polyomaviruses and papillomaviruses in prostatic tissue reveals the prostate as a habitat for multiple viral infections, *Prostate* 53 (2002): 263–276.

22. H. D. Strickler, R. Burk, K. Shah, et al., A multifaceted study of human papillomavirus and prostate carcinoma, *Cancer* 82 (1998): 1118–25; H.-O. Adami, H. Kuper, S.-O. Andersson, et al., Prostate cancer risk and serologic evidence of human papilloma virus infection: A population-based case-control study, *Cancer Epidemiology, Biomarkers, and Prevention* 12 (2003): 872–875.

23. Patrick C. Walsh and Janet F. Worthington, *Dr. Patrick Walsh's Guide to Surviving Prostate Cancer* (New York: Time Warner, 2001), 76.

24. P. Scardino and J. Kelman, *Dr. Peter Scardino's Prostate Book: The Complete Guide to Overcoming Prostate Cancer, Prostatitis, and BPH* (New York: Avery, 2005), 119.

25. L. K. Dennis and D. V. Dawson, Meta-analysis of measures of sexual activity and prostate cancer, *Epidemiology* 13 (2002): 72–79; L. Fernandez, Y. Galán, R. Jiménez, et al., Sexual behaviour, history of sexually transmitted diseases, and the risk of prostate cancer: A case-control study in Cuba, *International Journal of Epidemiology* 34 (2005): 193–197; N. Lightfoot, M. Conlon, N. Kreiger, et al., Medical history, sexual, and maturational factors and prostate cancer risk, *Annals of Epidemiology* 14 (2004): 655–662; K. A. Rosenblatt, K. G. Wicklund, and J. L. Stanford, Sexual factors and the risk of prostate cancer, *American Journal of Epidemiology* 153 (2001): 1152–58; M. L. Taylor, A. G. Mainous III, and B. J. Wells, Prostate cancer and sexually transmitted diseases: A meta-analysis, *Family Medicine* 37 (2005): 506–512.

26. L. K. Dennis, J. M. Ritchie, and M. I. Resnick, Prostate cancer and consistency of reporting sexual histories in men over age 50, *Prostate Cancer and Prostatic Diseases* 8 (2005): 243–247.

27. R. K. Ross, D. M. Deapen, J. T. Casagrande, et al., A cohort study of mortality from cancer of the prostate in Catholic priests, *British Journal of Cancer* 43 (1981): 233–235.

28. A. W. Hsing, Hormones and prostate cancer: What's next? *Epidemiologic Reviews* 23 (2001): 42–58. See also F. D. Gaylis, D. W. Lin, J. M. Ignatoff, et al., Prostate cancer in men using testosterone supplementation, *Journal of*

Urology 174 (2005): 534–538; and E. L. Rhoden and A. Morgentaler, Risks of testosterone-replacement therapy and recommendations for monitoring, *New England Journal of Medicine* 350 (2004): 482–492.

29. L. Ellis and H. Nyborg, Racial/ethnic variations in male testosterone levels: A probable contributor to group differences in health, *Steroids* 57 (1992): 72–75; R. Ross, L. Bernstein, R. A. Lobo, et al., 5-alpha-reductase activity and risk of prostate cancer among Japanese and US white and black males, *Lancet* 339 (1992): 887–889; I. Cheng, M. C. Yu, W.-P. Koh, et al., Comparison of prostate-specific antigen and hormone levels among men in Singapore and the United States, *Cancer Epidemiology, Biomarkers, and Prevention* 14 (2005): 1692–96.

30. Walsh and Worthington, *Dr. Patrick Walsh's Guide*, 47.

31. B. Armstrong and R. Doll, Environmental factors and cancer incidence and mortality in different countries, with special reference to dietary practices, *International Journal of Cancer* 15 (1975): 617–631.

32. M. B. Veierod, P. Laake, and D. S. Thelle, Dietary fat intake and risk of prostate cancer: A prospective study of 25,708 Norwegian men, *International Journal of Cancer* 73 (1997): 634–638; L. N. Kolonel, A. M. Y. Nomura, and R. V. Cooney, Dietary fat and prostate cancer: Current status, *Journal of the National Cancer Institute* 91 (1999): 414–428.

33. K. Hickey, K.-A. Do, and A. Green, Smoking and prostate cancer, *Epidemiologic Reviews* 23 (2001): 115–125.

34. L. K. Dennis and R. B. Hayes, Alcohol and prostate cancer, *Epidemiologic Reviews* 23 (2001): 110–114.

35. E. Bernal-Delgado, J. Latour-Pérez, F. Pradas-Arnal, et al., The association between vasectomy and prostate cancer: A systematic review of the literature, *Fertility and Sterility* 70 (1998): 191–200.

36. V. N. Giri, A. E. Cassidy, J. Beebe-Dimmer, et al., Association between Agent Orange and prostate cancer: A pilot case-control study, *Journal of Urology* 63 (2004): 757–761.

37. V. Verougstraete and D. Lison, Cadmium, lung and prostate cancer: A systematic review of recent epidemiological data, *Journal of Toxicology and Environmental Health, Part B* 6 (2003): 227–255.

13. Factors That May Prevent Emergence or Recurrence

1. E. Giovannucci, E. B. Rimm, Y. Liu, et al., A prospective study of tomato products, lycopene, and prostate cancer risk, *Journal of the National Cancer Institute* 94 (2002): 391–398; E.-S. Hwang and P. E. Bowen, Can the consumption of tomatoes or lycopene reduce cancer risk? *Integrative Cancer Therapies* 1 (2002): 121–132.

2. Giovannucci et al., A prospective study.

3. M. Saleem, V. M. Adhami, I. A. Siddiqui, et al., Tea beverage in chemoprevention of prostate cancer: A mini-review, *Nutrition and Cancer* 47 (2003):

13–23; L. Jian, L. P. Xie, A. H. Lee, et al., Protective effect of green tea against prostate cancer: A case-control study in southeast China, *International Journal of Cancer* 108 (2004): 130–135.

4. M. J. Messina, Emerging evidence on the role of soy in reducing prostate cancer risk, *Nutrition Reviews* 61 (2003): 117–131; A. Hikosaka, M. Asamoto, N. Hokaiwado, et al., Inhibitory effects of soy isoflavones on rat prostate carcinogenesis induced by 2-amino-1-methyl-6-phenylimidazo[4,5-*b*]pyridine (PhIP), *Carcinogenesis* 25 (2004): 381–387; Messina, Emerging evidence; T. Sonoda, Y. Nagata, M. Mori, et al., A case-control study of diet and prostate cancer in Japan: Possible protective effect of traditional Japanese diet, *Cancer Science* 95 (2004): 238–242.

5. W. M. Schoonen, C. A. Salinas, L. A. L. M. Kiemeney, et al., Alcohol consumption and risk of prostate cancer in middle-aged men, *International Journal of Cancer* 113 (2005): 133–140.

6. C. Pelucchi, R. Talamini, C. Galeone, et al., Fibre intake and prostate cancer risk, *International Journal of Cancer* 109 (2004): 278–280.

7. J. H. Cohen, A. R. Kristal, and J. L. Stanford, Fruit and vegetable intakes and prostate cancer, *Journal of the National Cancer Institute* 92 (2000): 61–68.

8. O. P. Heinonen, D. Albanes, J. Virtamo, et al., Prostate cancer and supplementation with alpha-tocopherol and beta-carotene: Incidence and mortality in a controlled trial, *Journal of the National Cancer Institute* 90 (1998): 440–446; E. Giovannucci, Gamma-tocopherol: A new player in prostate cancer prevention? (editorial), *Journal of the National Cancer Institute* 92 (2000): 1966–67; K. J. Helzlsouer, H.-Y. Huang, A. J. Alberg, et al., Association between alpha-tocopherol, gamma-tocopherol, selenium, and subsequent prostate cancer, *Journal of the National Cancer Institute* 92 (2000): 2018–23.

9. E. Giovannucci, A. Ascherio, E. B. Rimm, et al., Intake of carotenoids and retinol in relation to risk of prostate cancer, *Journal of the National Cancer Institute* 87 (1995): 1767–76; G. Bjelakovic, D. Nikolova, R. G. Simonetti, et al., Antioxidant supplements for prevention of gastrointestinal cancers: A systematic review and meta-analysis, *Lancet* 364 (2004): 1219–28.

10. C. Vanchieri, Studies shedding light on vitamin D and cancer, *Journal of the National Cancer Institute* 96 (2004): 735–736. See also E. M. John, G. G. Schwartz, J. Koo, et al., Sun exposure, vitamin D receptor gene polymorphisms, and risk of advanced prostate cancer, *Cancer Research* 65 (2005): 5470–79.

11. B. Higgins and I. M. Thompson, The prostate cancer prevention trial: Current status, *Journal of Urology* 171 (2004): S15–S18; A. Zuger, A big study yields big questions, *New England Journal of Medicine* 349 (2003): 213–214.

12. J. Shannon, S. Tewoderos, M. Garzotto, et al., Statins and prostate cancer risk: A case-control study, *American Journal of Epidemiology* 162 (2005): 318–325; M. S. Cyrus-David, A. Weinberg, T. Thompson, et al., The effect of

statins on serum prostate specific antigen levels in a cohort of airline pilots: A preliminary report, *Journal of Urology* 173 (2005): 1923–25; K. M. Dale, C. I. Coleman, N. N. Henyen, et al., Statins and cancer risk: A meta-analysis, *Journal of the American Medical Association* 295 (2006): 74–80.

13. S. Mahmud, E. Franco, and A. Aprikian, Prostate cancer and use of nonsteroidal anti-inflammatory drugs: Systematic review and meta-analysis, *British Journal of Cancer* 90 (2004): 93–99; E. J. Jacobs, C. Rodriguez, A. M. Mondul, et al., A large cohort study of aspirin and other nonsteroidal anti-inflammatory drugs and prostate cancer incidence, *Journal of the National Cancer Institute* 97 (2005): 975–980.

14. I.-M. Lee, H. D. Sesso, J.-J. Chen, et al., Does physical activity play a role in the prevention of prostate cancer? *Epidemiologic Reviews* 23 (2001): 132–137; C. M. Friedenreich, S. E. McGregor, K. S. Courneya, et al., Case-control study of lifetime total physical activity and prostate cancer risk, *American Journal of Epidemiology* 159 (2004): 740–749; A. V. Patel, C. Rodriguez, E. J. Jacobs, et al., Recreational physical activity and risk of prostate cancer in a large cohort of U.S. men, *Cancer Epidemiology, Biomarkers, and Prevention* 14 (2005): 275–279; E. L. Giovannucci, Y. Liu, M. F. Leitzmann, et al., A prospective study of physical activity and incident and fatal prostate cancer, *Archives of Internal Medicine* 165 (2005): 1005–10.

15. S. J. Freedland, W. B. Isaacs, L. A. Mangold, et al., Stronger association between obesity and biochemical progression after radical prostatectomy among men treated in the last 10 years, *Clinical Cancer Research* 11 (2005): 2883–88; S. J. Freedland, E. A. Platz, J. C. Presti, et al., Obesity, serum prostate specific antigen and prostate size, *Journal of Urology* 175 (2006): 500–4; M. P. Porter and J. L. Stanford, Obesity and the risk of prostate cancer, *Prostate* 62 (2005): 316–321.

16. D. Ornish, G. Weidner, W. R. Fair, et al., Intensive lifestyle changes may affect the progression of prostate cancer, *Journal of Urology* 174 (2005): 1065–70.

14. Science and Politics

1. C. Leaf, Why we're losing the war on cancer (and how to win it), *Fortune*, March 22, 2004, 77ff.

2. Ibid.

3. *A Review of the Department of Defense's Program for Breast Cancer Research* (Washington, D.C.: National Academy Press, 1997), vi–vii.

4. C. Daniels, The man who changed medicine, *Fortune*, November 29, 2004, 90ff.

5. Leon Jaroff, The man's cancer, *Time*, April 1, 1996.

6. Daniels, The man who changed medicine.

7. U.S. Senate adopts resolution encouraging doctors to inform prostate cancer patients about all proven treatments, *Business Wire*, October 13, 2004.

8. J. Strax, Lupron kickbacks betrayed prostate cancer patient trust, February 27, 2001, http://psa-rising.com/upfront/lupron-scam-mar01.htm, accessed October 6, 2005; Associated Press, TAP to pay $150m to settle Lupron suits, November 30, 2004.

15. Advice for Men Who Do Not Have Prostate Cancer

1. S. J. Jacobsen, E. J. Bergstralh, S. K. Katusic, et al., Screening digital rectal examination and prostate cancer mortality: A population-based case-control study, *Urology* 52 (1998): 173–179; S. Weinmann, K. Richert-Boe, A. G. Glass, et al., Prostate cancer screening and mortality: A case-control study (United States), *Cancer Causes and Control* 14 (2004): 133–138.

2. G. Bartsch, W. Horninger, H. Klocker, et al., Prostate cancer mortality after introduction of prostate-specific antigen mass screening in the Federal State of Tyrol, Austria, *Urology* 58 (2001): 417–424.

3. J. Concato, C. K. Wells, R. I. Horwitz, et al., The effectiveness of screening for prostate cancer, *Archives of Internal Medicine* 166 (2006): 38–43; M. J. Barry, The PSA conundrum, *Archives of Internal Medicine* 166 (2006): 7–8; J. K. Gohagan, P. C. Prorok, R. B. Hayes, et al., The Prostate, Lung, Colorectal and Ovarian (PLCO) Cancer Screening Trial of the National Cancer Institute: History, organization, status, *Controlled Clinical Trials* 21 (2000): 251S–272S; F. H. Schröder and C. H. Bangma, The European Randomized Study of Screening for Prostate Cancer (ERSPC), *British Journal of Urology* 79 (suppl. 1) (1997): 68–71.

4. T. A. Stamey, M. Caldwell, J. E. McNeal, et al., The prostate specific antigen era in the United States is over for prostate cancer: What happened in the last 20 years? *Journal of Urology* 172 (2004): 1297–1301.

5. W. J. Catalona and S. Loeb, The PSA era is not over for prostate cancer, *European Urology* 48 (2005): 541–545.

6. Government panel: Benefit of prostate screening uncertain, American Cancer Society News Center, accessed on www.cancer.org., September 4, 2004.

7. Sheldon Marks, *Prostate and Cancer: A Family Guide to Diagnosis, Treatment, and Survival,* 3rd ed. (New York: Perseus, 2003), 68.

8. J. Fang, E. J. Metter, P. Landis, et al., Low levels of prostate-specific antigen predict long-term risk of prostate cancer: Results from the Baltimore Longitudinal Study of Aging, *Urology* 58 (2001): 411–416; P. H. Gann, C. H. Hennekens, and M. J. Stampfer, A prospective evaluation of plasma prostate-specific antigen for detection of prostatic cancer, *Journal of the American Medical Association* 273 (1995): 289–294.

9. A. S. Whittemore, P. M. Cirillo, D. Feldman, et al., Prostate specific antigen levels in young adulthood predict prostate cancer risk: Results from a cohort of black and white Americans, *Journal of Urology* 174 (2005): 872–876.

10. X. Wang, J. Yu, A. Sreekumar, et al., Autoantibody signatures in prostate cancer, *New England Journal of Medicine* 353 (2005): 1224–35.

11. C. Kumar-Sinha and A. M. Chinnaiyan, Molecular markers to identify patients at risk for recurrence after primary treatment for prostate cancer, *Urology* 62 (suppl. 6B) (2003): 19–35.

Appendix A. The Anatomy and Function of the Prostate Gland

1. Robert Hitchcock, *Love, Sex, and PSA* (San Diego: TMC Press, 1997), 62.

2. Peter T. Scardino and Judith Kelman, *Dr. Peter Scardino's Prostate Book: The Complete Guide to Overcoming Prostate Cancer, Prostatitis, and BPH* (New York: Avery, 2005), 30.

3. Bert Gottlieb and Thomas J. Mawn, *The Men's Club: How To Lose Your Prostate Without Losing Your Sense of Humor* (Oxnard, Calif.: Pathfinder Publishing, 1999), 11.

INDEX

abarelix, 68, 70–71
acupuncture, 81
Adamec, Christine, 150, 229
Adam's Burden (Neider), 3, 17,
    154, 230–31
  on bowel complications, 58
  on radiation treatment, 49
  on support groups, 131
adenocarcinomas, 11, 12
adjuvant therapy, 77, 155, 160
Affirming the Darkness (Wheeler
    and Wheeler), 121, 125, 150,
    165, 167, 234
African American men, 83, 171–
    73, 185, 214, 215, 234
age, 28, 42–43, 169, 170
  costs of treatment and, 108,
    109
  death and, 8–9, 90–91, 167
  diet and, 189
  genetics and, 175
  incidence of prostate cancer
    and, 169–70
  life expectancy and, 95–96
  metastasis rates and, 156
  onset of prostate cancer, 60,
    161, 225–27, 231–32, 234,
    239
  prostate enlargement and,
    219, 222

sexual activity and, 178–79
sexual function and, 142, 144,
    147, 149
testing and, 214, 215, 216
urinary function and, 40, 134
alcohol consumption, 183–84,
    192, 197
alendronate, 74
alternative therapies, 81–87
Alterowitz, Ralph and Barbara,
    146, 224
American Cancer Society, 5, 23,
    130–31, 200, 206
  testing recommendations of,
    214
  website, 238
American Society for Therapeu-
    tic Radiology and Oncology
    (ASTRO), 59, 60
American Urological Associa-
    tion, 110
Americans with Disabilities Act
    (1990), 129
Anandron, 70
Anderson Cancer Center, 105
anemia, 75, 165
anesthesia, 29, 32, 33, 34, 105
  cryotherapy and, 115
  radiation treatment and, 54
  seed therapy and, 51